LOW THIOL
recipes

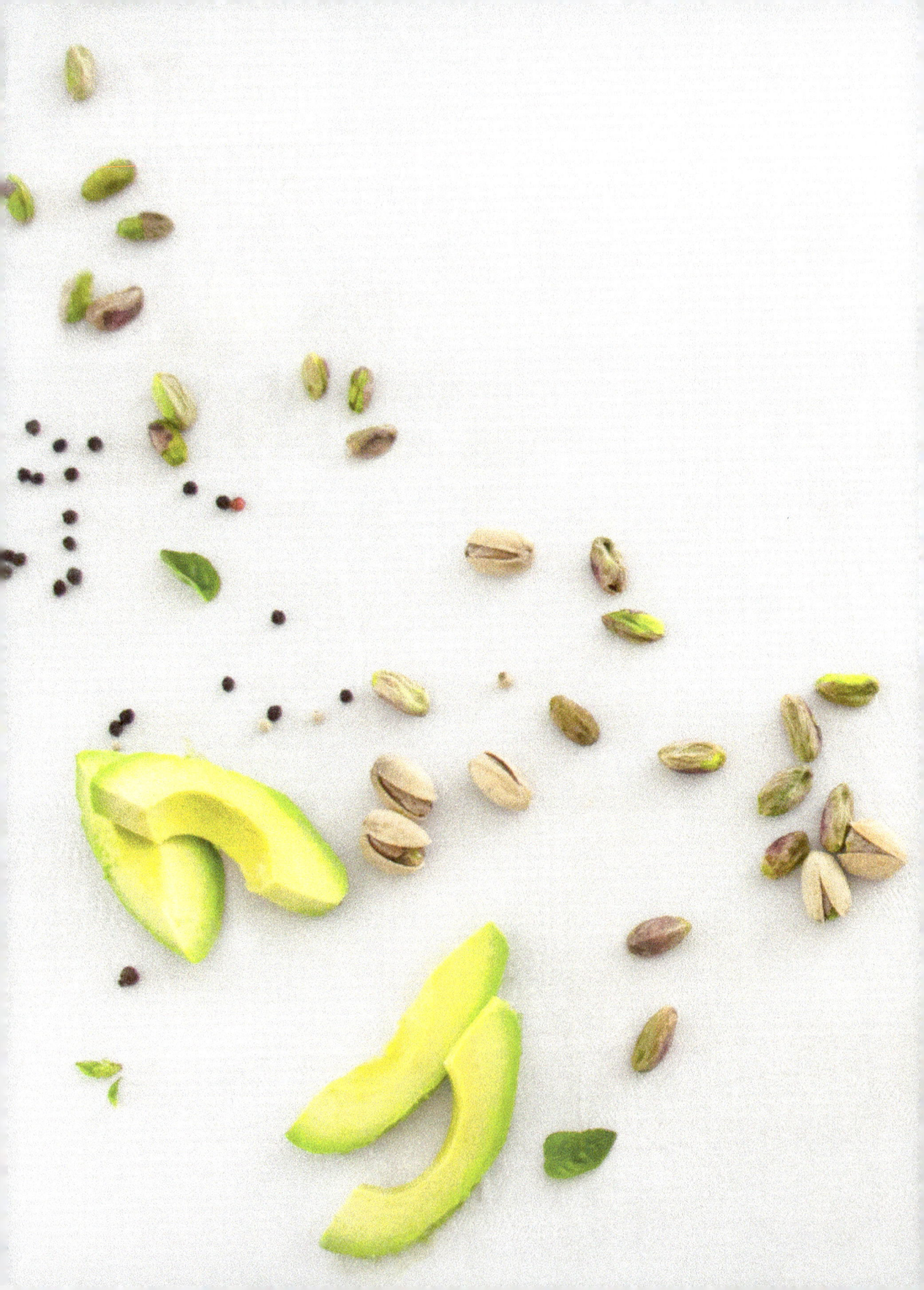

LOW THIOL
recipes

With over 70 low thiol recipes to improve your
physical & mental wellbeing

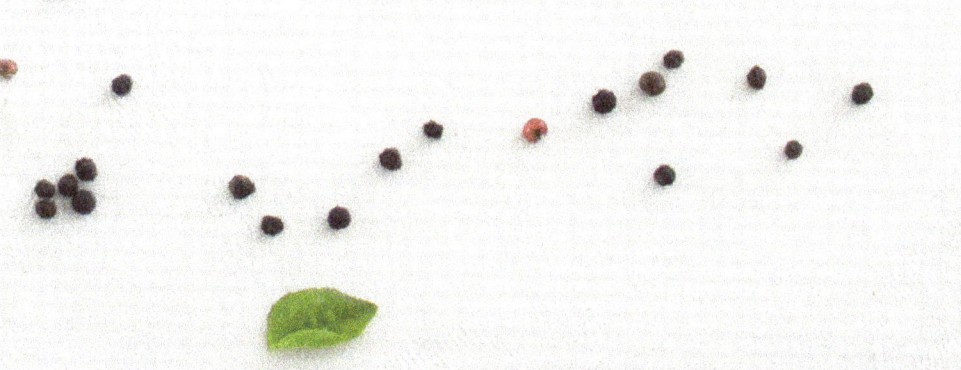

Jillaine Williams with Michelle Eady

forward by Joann Loos

The information contained in this book is provided for general and educational purposes only. It is not intended as nor does it replace medical advice. You the reader are encouraged to seek medical advice before embarking upon this or any dietary protocol. If you have health problems you should consult a qualified health or medical professional in relation to advice contained in this book.

The writer does not take any responsibility for any outcomes associated with the use of these recipes or protocols referred to in this book. It is the reader's responsibility to confirm that any information, products, foods, services and other information provided is appropriate for you.

Low Thiol Recipes: For symptoms of mercury toxicity and thiol intolerance

First published in Australia in 2019 by
Name: Jillaine K Williams
Address: 573 Wattle Grove Road,
Wattle Grove, Tasmania. 7109
T: +61407 403 787
First published in 2019 by
www.lowthiolrecipes.com

Copyright © 2019 Jillaine Kay Williams,

First Edition.
All rights reserved. No part of this publication may be reproduced, transmitted in any form by any means, electronic, mechanical, photocopying, recording or otherwise without permission in writing from the publisher.

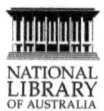

A catalogue record for this book is available from the National Library of Australia

Printed in Australia and USA
Title:
Low Thiol Recipes: A diet for mercury toxicity.

ISBN:
978-0-6485644-0-9 (paperback)
978-0-6485644-1-6 (ePub)

Notes:
    included index
Subjects:
    Detoxification (Health)
    Cooking (Natural Foods)
    Mercury toxicity
    Chelation

Photography:
    Jillaine Williams

Food Stylist:
    Michelle Eady
Design:
    Kate Doyle

Dedication

If your quality of life has been negatively impacted by mercury toxicity - this is for you in the hope that you may now find some relief.

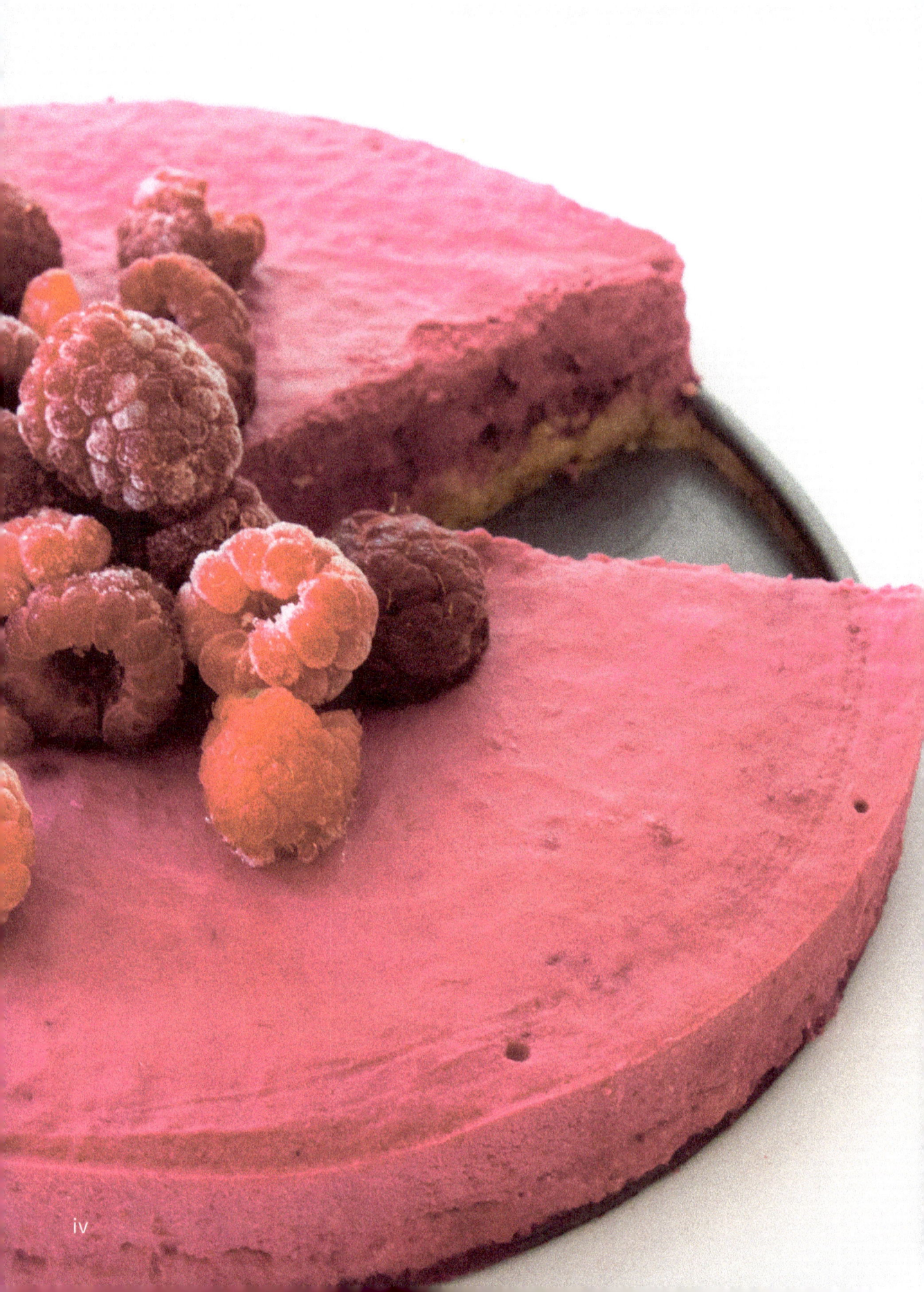

Acknowledgments

A wonderful twist of fate introduced me to local Tasmanian artist Michelle Eady. Michelle came to work with me and took enthusiastically to the task of researching recipes and applying her unquestionable food styling skills in our test kitchen. It is my hope that Michelle's keen artists' eye will be applied to many more biomed-style recipe books in the future.

Great friendships were developed during the many hours of cooking, photographing and dishwashing. Our precious Josie - acted as our tireless 'dish pig', ploughing through mountains of dishes without complaint.

Keeping abreast of nutritional research and development is one thing, however, producing a cook book adds a whole new level of demand upon relationships. As any natural health practitioner can tell you, the support of family is vital in a world that doesn't always see things our way. Daniel, Dylan, Emma, Emile, Sophia, Olivia and my dear-heart Rob - I love you all.

Thanks to my local Cygnet independent grocery store owner George for his assistance in sourcing some very unusual ingredients not normally stocked in downtown Cygnet. Much gratitude to Esther, our local Heartfelt Wholefoods store keeper.

To my friends Judy, Bridget, Danielle and Ginny for their love, recipe ideas and wealth of foodie experience, thank you.

Most importantly I wish to acknowledge the work of Dr Andy Cutler and the ongoing efforts of his widow Joann. Andy was accessible and generous with his time and knowledge. I will always feel honored to have known him and to have been inspired by him. Thank you, Joann for your ongoing kindness, support and for continuing to disseminate Andy's vital work.

Jillaine K Williams
Wattle Grove, Tasmania 2019

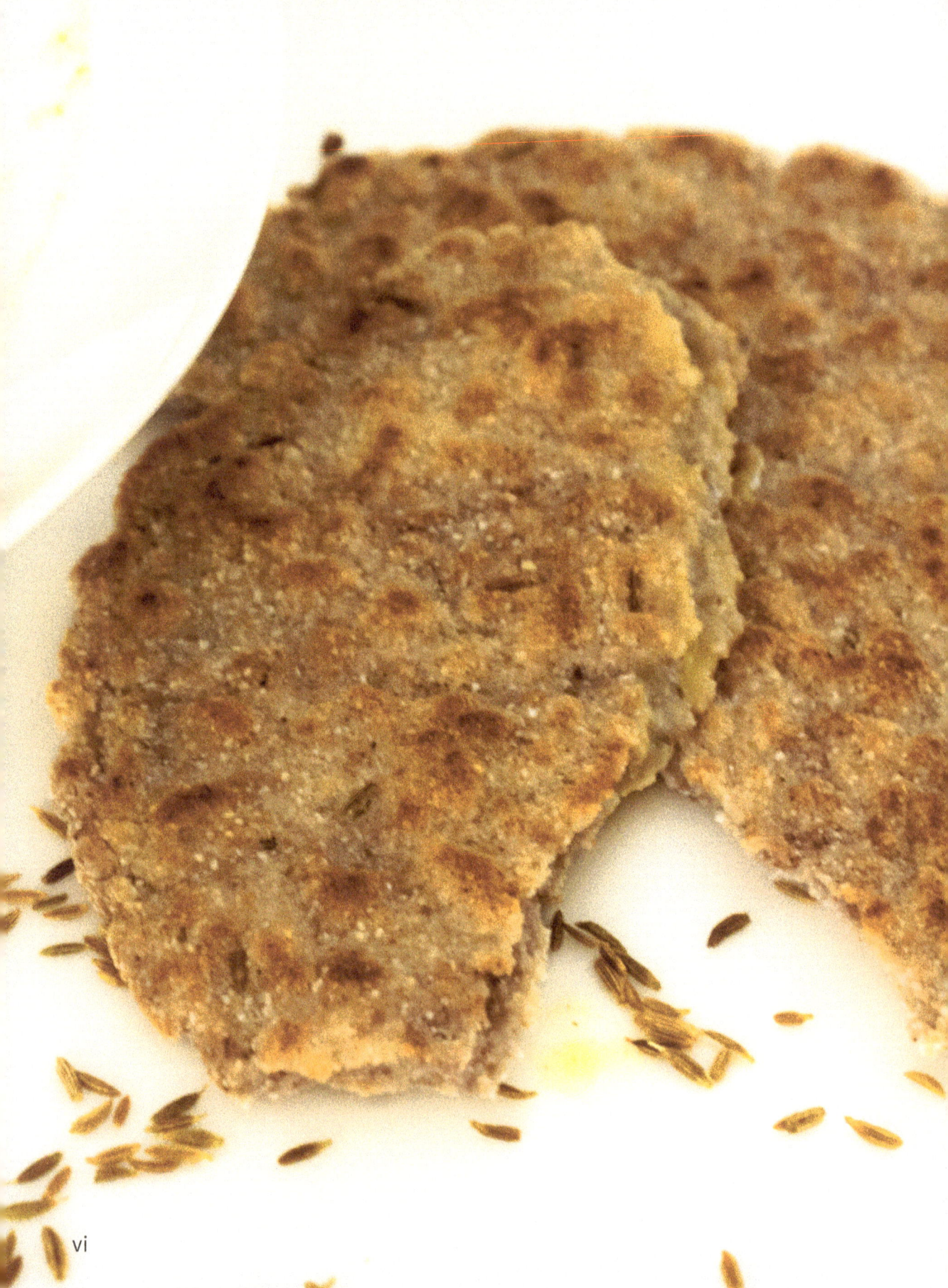

Forward by Joann Loos

As many of you know, Andy Cutler came up with the high and low thiol food lists. Here's the story of how that came about.

Andy was working as a consulting chemical engineer. While deep into one project, he was so engrossed he didn't want to go shopping and so ate only this wonderful bread from a local German bakery. He felt great and could concentrate on the project.

When that bread ran out, he went to the nearest grocery store and bought what he thought was an equivalent loaf of bread. While eating that loaf he felt tired and had trouble concentrating. Once that loaf was done, the bakery was open, so he got the good bread. He perked right up.

He went to talk to the baker. The baker described to him how mass-produced bread uses enzymes (usually whey) to help the bread rise faster and brown quicker. Andy researched whey and discovered that it contained thiols, a specific type of molecule that can move mercury around in the body, but not help get it out. That started him on his research of the food lists.

What you may not know was that he was very sensitive to thiols. So he tried all the foods out on the lists himself to determine if they were high or low thiol. If he reacted, the food was high thiol. I still have food he planned to try in our pantry.

This cookbook will give you some great recipes and ideas for low thiol cooking. Andy always made tasty food that met his dietary requirements and now you can too.

Joann Loos
Andy Cutler Publishing
noamalgam.com

HIGH Thiol foods

Foods to avoid

- cabbage
- bok choy
- coriander leaf
- turnips
- eggs
- asparagus
- dairy products, whey
- legumes
- chocolate
- brussels sprouts
- broccoli
- coffee
- the onion family
- kale
- cauliflower
- chlorella

This list is not exhaustive

The complete version can be found in
The Mercury Detoxification Manual- A guide to Mercury Chelation
by Rebecca Rust Lee and Andrew Hall Cutler PhD, PE

Further Reading and Resources

1. Andrew Hall Cutler (1999) *Amalgam Illness: Diagnosis and Treatment*. Andy Cutler Publishing, ISBN 978-0-9676168-3-4. noamalgam.com

2. Andrew Hall Cutler (2004) *Hair Test Interpretation: Finding Hidden Toxicities*. Andy Cutler Publishing, ISBN 978-0-9676168-2-7. noamalgam.com

3. Andrew Hall Cutler and Rebecca Rust Lee (2019) *The Mercury Detoxification Manual: A Guide to Mercury Chelation*. Andy Cutler Publishing, ISBN 978-0-9676168-4-1. noamalgam.com

4. David Olsen MD (2018) *Mercury Toxicity*. Available at https://emedicine.medscape.com/article/1175560-overview

5. Jillaine Williams. *Low Thiol Recipes*. Available at www.lowthiolrecipes.com

6. Metabiome DNA testing. *See Pantry Practitioner below*

7. Natural Resource Defense Council *Smart Seafood Buying Guide*. Available at www.nrdc.org/stories/mercury-guide

8. Pantry Practitioner. *Nutrition consultancy, hair test and interpretation service*. www.pantrypractitioner.com.au/ jillaine@pantrypractitioner.com.au

9. Sara Russell and Kristin Homme. *Mercury as Antinutrient*. Wise Traditions In Food, Farming and the Healing Arts. The Weston A. Price Foundation, Volume 19 Number 1, Spring (2018) Available at www.westonaprice.org/journal-spring-2018-mercury-toxicity/

10. Sylvia Onusic. *Poisoning Our Children. Wise Traditions In Food, Farming and the Healing Arts*. The Weston A. Price Foundation, Volume 19 Number 1, Spring (2018) Available at www.westonaprice.org/journal-spring-2018-mercury-toxicity/

11. Weston A. Price Foundation: for wise traditions in food, farming and the healing arts; on-line journals and articles www.westonaprice.org/

Groups and Support

Andy Cutler Chelation: Safe Mercury and Heavy Metal Detox Facebook Group
www.facebook.com/groups/acfanatics

ACC for Parents Facebook Group
www.facebook.com/groups/ACCforParents/

Low Thiol Recipes Facebook Group
www.facebook.com/groups/492609177997602/

Weston A. Price Facebook Group
www.facebook.com/westonaprice/

Ingredients and Stockists

Please see our web site for updates on stockists in your area.
www.lowthiolrecipebook.com

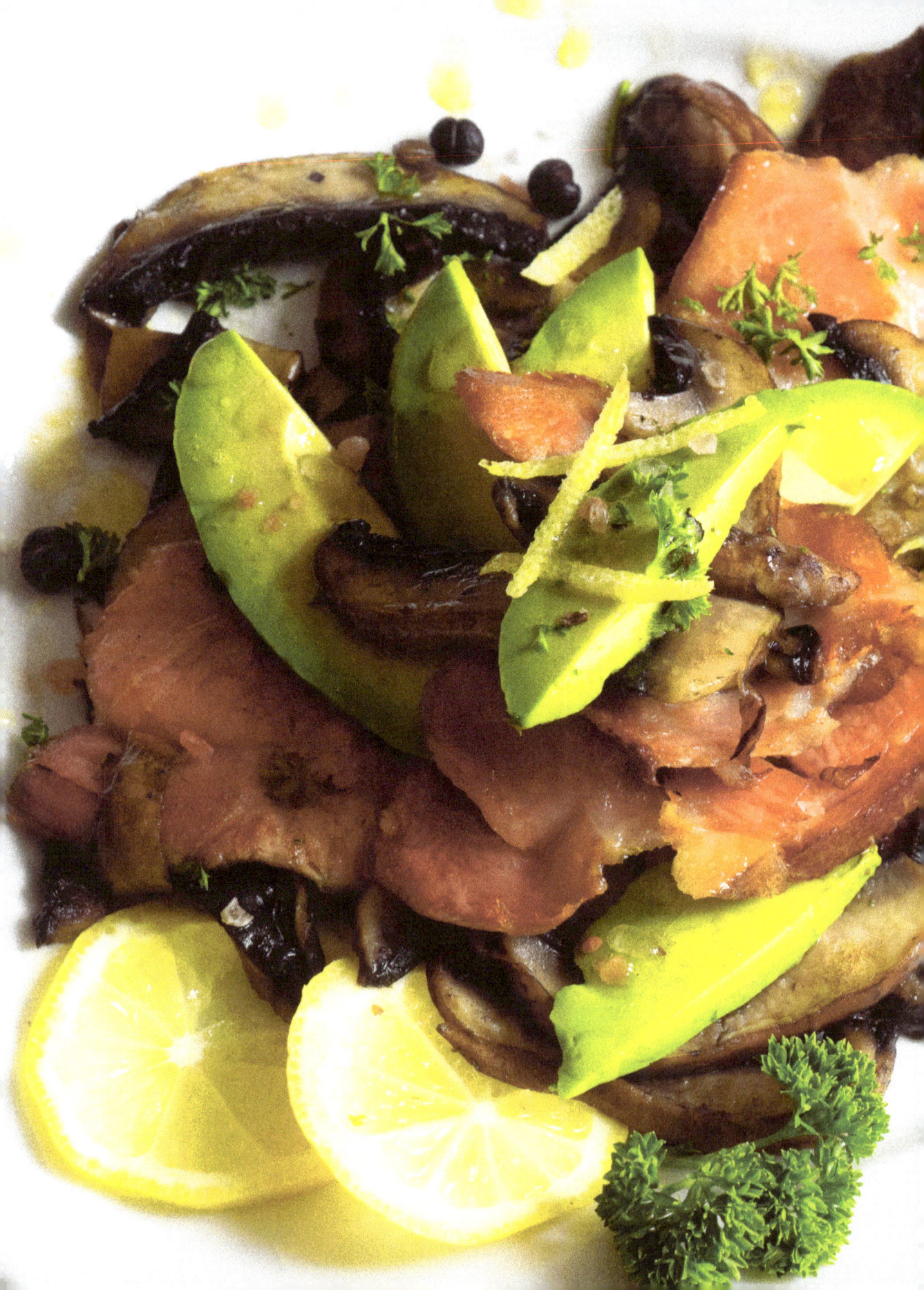

Contents

Acknowledgments — v
Forward by Joann Loos — vii
High Thiol Foods — viii
Further Reading and Resources — ix
Introduction — xii
The importance of your microbiota — xx
Grains, legumes, nuts and seeds — xxiv
Symbol Key — xxviii
Baking Conversion Charts — xxix

Rise & Shine — 1

A Little Something on the side — 13

Warm Your Heart Soups — 31

The Main Attraction — 37

I'm Just Too Tired To Cook! — 57

You're Sweet Enough — 65

The Way To My Heart — 73

Bevvies & Brews & Condiments — 89

Index — 101

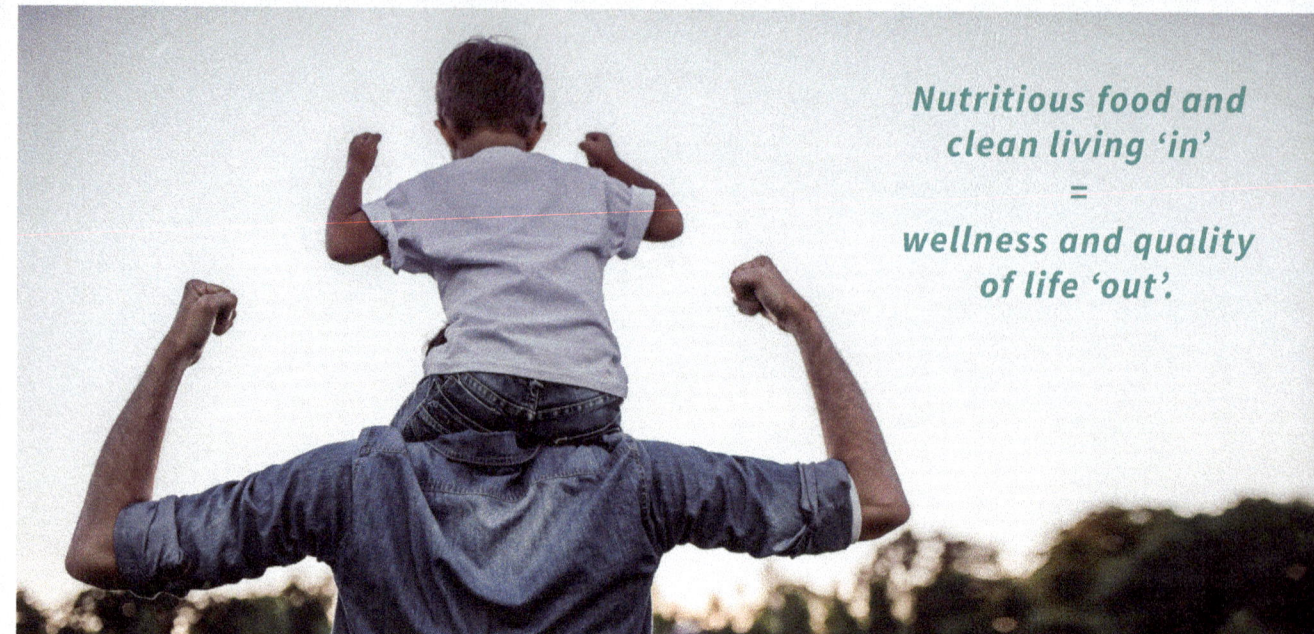

Nutritious food and clean living 'in'

=

wellness and quality of life 'out'.

Introduction

Looking for pieces to a puzzle - is industry driving an increase in chronic disease?

I felt compelled from a young age to study nutritional medicine in order to gain a deeper understanding of the cause and effects of industrialised foods upon our health. Having witnessed first hand the different health outcomes for people raised on whole foods in a rural setting, such as my mother and subsequent generations, granted access to processed and convenience foods, such as my generation. It seemed pretty straight forward to me at the time.

The past decade however has seen a steep increase in chronic illness in both children and adults. I notice in my own practice that clients present with health concerns of an increasingly complex nature. People with multi-system disorders from adrenal and thyroid hormone disturbances, through gut and immune issues to difficulties with brain, mood and memory function.

It is no longer sufficient it seems to optimise the diet or support biochemical pathways using natural medicines or to encourage lifestyle changes as important as these are. I often felt disappointed in treatment outcomes when using these approaches in isolation. A piece of the puzzle was missing. The holistic approach to finding and addressing 'the cause' of this rise in chronic disease although effective in many cases does not always provide all the pieces. Advances made in integrative pathology testing I believe reflects this dilemma.

The following is just a sample of how testing has evolved in our quest for answers.

- **Nutrigenomics profiling:** The term nutrigenomics brings together nutrients and genetics. Research in the area of human genomics demonstrates that diet and nutrients can alter the way your genes function and therefore your health outcomes. We're looking to genetics to help tailor nutritional support.

- **Gut microbiome testing:** we can get a clear picture via stool testing of the vast communities of microbes, fungi, archaea and viruses living in our gut. More and more research is revealing the impact of our gut bugs upon many aspects of health. Even mental health can be impacted by an unbalanced bug population.

- **Mold exposure, sick building and toxin evaluations:** testing for mold, biotoxins and chemical exposure can help to determine if your home or environment is contributing to illness. This form of testing is relevant now as our exposure to organophosphates, volatile solvents, PCBs, pesticides and plastics has become widespread.

- **Screening for increasingly virulent infectious diseases, super bugs, viruses:** an era of medical dependence upon antibiotics and its widespread use in our food supply has resulted in less resistance to infection and a reduced effectiveness of standard treatments.

- **An assortment of additional functional pathology testing** such as hormone profiling to assess the impact of stress and nutrient deficiencies, markers of inflammation to assess immune system dysregulation, allergy and intolerance profiling to assess individual sensitivities and more.

- **Heavy metal evaluation via hair, urine, blood and stool: we've** known since the industrial revolution of the potential for toxic metals to do harm. Commonly though these reports have failed to deliver usable information.

Even with valuable tools such as these, it seems the majority of health care practitioners continue to overlook a crucial piece to the puzzle.

That piece for me, was discovering the extensive works of Andrew (Andy) Hall Cutler PhD. Reading his books and having conversations with Andy brought home the critical importance of the wide spread effects of mercury, it's impact on multiple body systems, and more importantly a safe method for removing it from the body as opposed to redistributing it and potentially causing more harm.[1]

I also learned that there are a number of markers which often turn up on a blood panel that may actually be pointing to mercury toxicity. This common pattern can provide another piece of the puzzle when we know what we are looking for.

- increased red blood cell size
- iron-deficiency anaemia which proves resistant to treatment
- elevated free-copper
- low blood sugar levels
- hormone imbalances with paradoxical control hormone levels
- low immune markers

This list is not exhaustive[2]

> **The majority of health care practitioners continue to overlook a crucial piece to the puzzle**

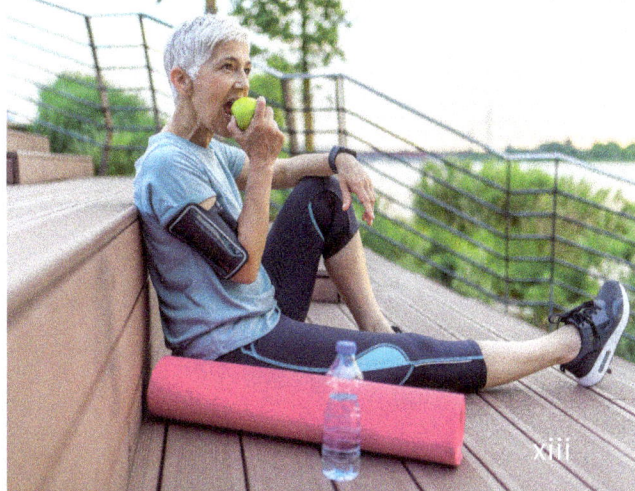

---

1. Andy Cutler's approach to chelation goes beyond the scope of this book however it can be found in his books in the resource section.
2. *Amalgam Illness: Diagnosis and Treatment* by Dr A Cutler. 1999 See Resource Section

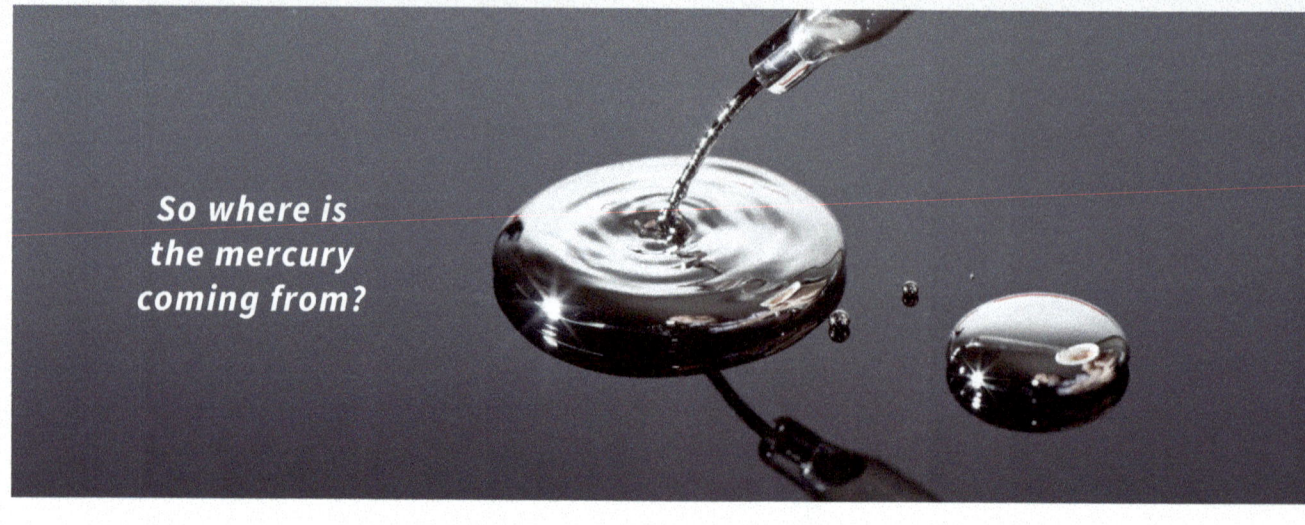

So where is the mercury coming from?

These markers should be a red flag for us as practitioners however they're commonly overlooked. This can put a patient on a long and expensive journey from one practitioner to another to treat their gut, their genes, their deficiencies and their inflammation without ever really getting to the main causative factor. Patients themselves often wind up frustrated and disappointed.

There is an ever-present risk that we will settle (once again) for treating the symptoms rather than identifying the primary cause.

I must give credit where credit is due and recognise the relatively few practitioners, trained in nutritional and environmental medicine, who do agree that the 'heavy metal' piece of the puzzle is important and are giving it their attention. They are thinking about mercury in their patients with complex issues and in some cases treating heavy metal poisoning. What appears to divide this group however is the approach to testing, interpreting and treating mercury toxicity. More on this later.

Mercury a closer look

The physiological impacts of mercury on the body is analogous to throwing a box full of spanners into a precision clock-work piece. The resulting impact is systemic and cumulative with perhaps the greatest damage being on the central nervous system and brain function. Mercury from all sources is poisonous to humans. The majority of health practitioners however are not considering mercury in their evaluation so it's hardly surprising that those adversely affected by mercury find themselves searching far and wide for answers and are often referred for mental health treatment. You have likely heard the term 'mad as a hatter' used to describe the symptoms of workers in the felt hat industry of the 19th century.

What does mercury toxicity look like?

Disease conditions from leaky gut to hormone and thyroid issues, mental health, cardiovascular disorders, immune and autoimmune disorders, cancer, chronic fatigue, attention deficit and autistic spectrum disorders, skin, joint and muscle issues all can be traced to the devastating impact of toxic metals and mercury in the body. One of the most notable symptoms of mercury poisoning however is erethism which presents as shyness, apathy and depression.

Mercury toxicity can and does present a complex clinical picture. From a holistic perspective we should be looking to find the cause of what ails us and to limit our exposure where possible.

Toxic exposure begins early

The toxic effects of mercury can begin before birth due to its capacity to damage gene function in either parent thus impacting a resulting fetus. The susceptibility of a developing fetus to mercury's neurotoxic effect results as mercury crosses the placenta, enters the fetal blood supply and subsequently crosses into the brain and central nervous system. Maternal exposure might include a diet high in longer-lived fish species, the introduction of flu vaccination during pregnancy, processed foods and environmental sources.

The 20th century brought not only food additives, processed and refined foods to the table, it brought new chemicals and toxic metals into our agricultural, medical and dental practices and into our homes in ever increasing variety.

Like most of my generation I had my teeth filled as a child with amalgam fillings no doubt attributable to the effects of the previously mentioned, modern, processed diet. What I soon learned is that these fillings contain 50% metallic mercury by weight and release a mercury vapor over the filling's lifetime. Once mercury finds its way into cells and tissue it can be notoriously difficult to remove as it has the capacity to disturb essential mineral transport and to increase the accumulation of other toxic metals. Small, repetitive exposures over time can therefore become a significant problem as toxic metals accumulate and lead to health conditions of a chronic nature.

Toxic exposure through the loss of gut integrity

At the same time as this increased environmental exposure to mercury we've also seen an increase in the use of antibiotics and glyphosate in the food chain contributing to a loss of microbial diversity, gut integrity and barrier function. Disruption of this important interface, between our inner and outer world, contributes to the uptake of toxins into the body via the gastrointestinal tract. As metals bio-accumulate in seafoods and in humans this appears to be the perfect storm.

No one case will look the same

Toxic exposure and genetic susceptibility.

You may be thinking "not everyone exposed to vaccines, amalgams or air pollution becomes chronically ill", and you would be right of course.

It's here that the science of human genomics comes into play. Our more recent ability to map our personal genome can help to identify those amongst us who are more vulnerable than others. The more relevant research findings can give us insights into an individuals' reduced detoxification capacity and an increased susceptibility to oxidative stress.[3] This has the effect of leaving a significant proportion of the population more susceptible to the damaging effects of these toxins. No one case will look the same, as a result of these contributing factors: exposure, age, genetics, microbial population and more importantly an individual's nutritional and antioxidant[4] status.

---

3 Oxidative stress is akin to rusting on a cellular level as heavy metals generate free radical or unbalanced molecules inside the body.

4 There are a variety of whole, natural foods which are rich in antioxidant nutrients including vitamins A, D, E, C, Selenium and plant-based phytonutrients. Antioxidant nutrients lessen the effects of free radicals.

Heavy metals as opportunistic elements

Heavy metals displace and antagonise the functions of essential elements in the body. It's for this reason that being heavy metal poisoned has such a broad spectrum of symptoms and disorders. Consider the hundreds of metabolic functions of zinc alone- growth, immune function, hormone and reproductive health. Knowing that mercury has a high affinity for zinc binding sites in the body, we begin to understand its potential to impact so many systems.

Similarly, being deficient in minerals such as zinc, calcium, iron or selenium will exacerbate your susceptibility to heavy metal toxicity. With both elements at play- the modern processed food diet and an increasing level of exposure there is little reason not to suspect heavy metals as contributors to our increasing rates of chronic disease.

Thiols- what are they and what do they have to do with mercury?

I have long been aware of natural substances for chelating or binding and escorting mercury from the body. I had recommended and tried them myself whilst my mercury-rich, amalgam fillings were still in place in my teeth. I couldn't understand why supplements containing chlorella or alpha lipoic acid or glutathione might make me feel worse when these supplements had been touted as being beneficial for metal detoxification. I felt more fatigued, brain fogged and headachy.

Further research into the nature of thiols has provided a better understanding of why some supplements might have this adverse effect where mercury is also in the mix. When I look now at the many detoxification protocols becoming available, I find that most authors and researchers are not offering satisfactory or safe solutions for the removal of this disruptive toxin from the body.

Why?

Because they're not considering the impact of free thiol containing foods and supplements in a mercury toxic and genetically susceptible body.

Monothiol   **Dithiol**

The following are a few facts to consider.

- A Thiol is a sulfur compound[5] which occurs in many foods including garlic, onion, cabbage, coffee, chocolate, beans, chlorella and coriander leaf.

- All are foods that we're encouraged to consume as part of a healing diet.

- Thiols are also present in supplements such as broccoli sprout powder, N-acetyl-cysteine (NAC) and Glutathione (GSH)- again commonly prescribed supplements for detoxification and health.

- Thiols are also known as mercaptans a term derived from the Latin mercurium captāns or 'capturing mercury' due to their affinity for and binding to Mercury (Hg).

- Thiols can be mono-thiol or di-thiol meaning that they have one or two metal binding sites respectively.[6]

Thiols are also known as mercaptans a term derived from the Latin mercurium captāns or 'capturing mercury' due to their affinity for and binding to Mercury (Hg)

Free Thiols - how do they cause symptoms?

At first the thiols' affinity for mercury seems beneficial however free thiols in food and supplements are mono-thiols and as such their bond with mercury is not a strong one and only serves to redistribute mercury around the body causing symptoms typical of heavy metal poisoning.

Knowing that the thiol-containing amino acid, cysteine, is abundant in protein structures inside the body helps to explain the mechanism by which damage occurs. Mercury binds to cysteine in tissues, enzymes, neurons and mitochondria causing a wide range of symptoms and disarray earning its reputation as the most toxic and damaging metal known to man.

Free thiols in foods and supplements are like a bus hurtling around inside the body with mercury as the high-jacker at the wheel. Cysteine is like an intricate power grid throughout the body which is being damaged by an out of control bus resulting in fires, loss of energy supply, structural damage and a broken transport system. You can expect to feel unwell with so much system-wide disruption.

It's for this reason that a low thiol diet for many relieves the symptoms of heavy metal toxicity including brain fog and fatigue.

The Low Thiol Diet as a simple way to investigate the likelihood of mercury toxicity

What if mercury is driving a break down in multiple biological systems in complex and chronic illness cases? What if a low thiol trial and hair analysis were the very first tests administered as a priority?

For around half of those with health conditions related to mercury exposure the low thiol diet can be an effective clinical tool to assess the likelihood that mercury is in fact contributing to their symptoms and underlying disease state.[7] If after a 10 day trial of the low-thiol diet followed by a rapid reintroduction of these foods you feel a distinct contrast in overall energy level and mental clarity you might then consider further investigations into mercury toxicity.

What else might I expect on a low thiol trial?

There are a number of symptoms which have been associated with mercury exposure and may be exacerbated by thiol-rich foods and supplements.

Whilst avoiding thiol-rich foods look for changes or improvements in any of the following areas.

- gastrointestinal disorders
- diarrhoea
- reduced cognitive function (fuzzy brain)
- depression

---

5 Free thiols differ from elemental sulfur found in a variety of foods.
6 The metal binding site on a thiol is called a sulfhydryl group and is made up of a sulfur atom bonded to a hydrogen atom, represented as -SH
7 Hair Test Interpretation: Finding Hidden Toxicities by Dr A Cutler. 2004 See the resource section.

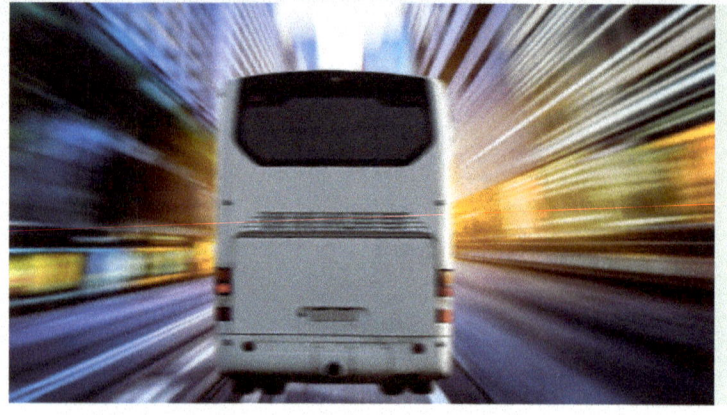

Free thiols in foods and supplements are like a bus hurtling around inside the body with mercury as the high-jacker at the wheel.

- tremor, nervous system disorders
- hormone disturbances including reproductive, thyroid and adrenal hormones
- yeast overgrowth
- a deep and often debilitating fatigue
- immune and autoimmune conditions

Dietary thiols don't affect everyone (with mercury burden) in the same way- this depends upon their body's level of sulfur amino acids, including cysteine, which in excess may lead to excitotoxicity, damage to neurons and vessels as well as those symptoms described above.

The list of thiol containing foods is extensive, therefore the diet can be quite restrictive. Particularly for those who have additional food intolerances.

Most importantly the Sulfur compounds found in these foods are essential to health in the long term so that a low thiol diet should ideally be supervised by a health professional and undertaken;

1. As a short-term trial (10 - 14 days) to determine if is helpful. If you do feel a marked improvement in symptoms, then this points to mercury toxicity and warrants further investigation.
2. To reduce the symptoms of heavy metals whilst taking measures to reduce the body burden of mercury so that these foods might eventually be returned to the diet.
3. The diet should not be continued if there is no notable improvements in cognitive and energy function.

The thiols' affinity for mercury seems beneficial however free thiols in food and supplements are mono-thiols and as such their bond with mercury is not a strong one and only serves to redistribute mercury around the body causing symptoms typical of heavy metal poisoning.

What is a chelator? Chelating metals safely out of the body to restore function.

The fact that you are reading this introduction suggests that you are well on your way to investigating and addressing any heavy metal issues you or your loved ones may be suffering. Here are a few guidelines which you may find helpful.

- A chelator is a molecule with two or more thiol groups and thus binds mercury and other metals extremely tightly to escort them out of the body. Please take advantage of our resource section to learn more about safe, low-dose methods of chelation.

- Trial a low-thiol diet to see if it positively impacts your symptoms.[8]

- Know that some people need more thiols and sulfur-rich foods in their diet. For them removing all high thiol foods will likely make them feel worse not better. For other thiols won't make much difference either way.

- Seek the support of a functional medicine or natural health practitioner who is familiar with the 'Cutler Chelation Protocol'.

- Note that recommendations to use chlorella, coriander, or thiol-rich supplements NAC, Glutathione and alpha lipoic acid may have the potential to do harm.

- A good deal of caution and care is required when addressing the removal of mercury.

> *A low thiol diet is NOT FOR EVERYONE with mercury poisoning. Some people need more thiols and sulfur-rich foods in their diet.*

- Seek out a 'biological' or integrative dentist to assess your amalgam fillings and to remove them safely if you so choose.

- Hair mineral analysis is a good place to begin by revealing patterns of disordered mineral transport and accumulation of toxic metals. Where there is mercury there is commonly additional heavy metal accumulation as mercury disrupts the transportation and detoxification systems in the body.[9]

---

8 Details of food lists can be found in The Mercury Detoxification Manual listed in the resource section.
9 For test and interpret services see the resource section.

I sincerely hope that a low-thiol protocol helps you to find the symptom relief that has eluded you to date.

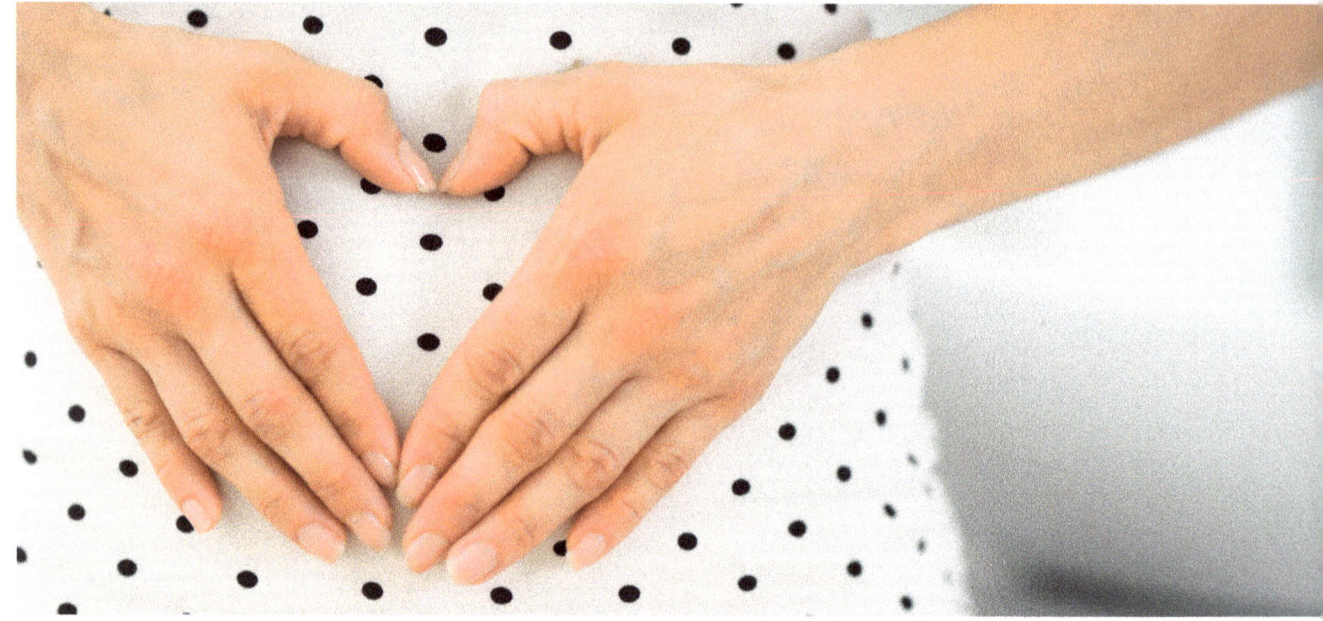

The importance of your microbiota and a nutrient-dense diet

There are a number of nutrients and food elements which can be useful when addressing heavy metal toxicity. Here are a few that I've found helpful.

Foods which support a healthy microbial population

This book includes fermented vegetables and fiber-rich foods to enable the building of a healthy bug population. Avoid chlorinated and fluoridated water and consult a Metabiome registered health care practitioner for an in-depth DNA based assessment of your microbiota. Restoring a healthy microbial balance in the digestive tract will in turn reduce your uptake of heavy metals.

Source organic and chemical free produce and products where possible

Reducing the toxic burden on our bodies requires that we address the source of those toxins. Whether it be amalgam fillings, food additives, cleaning products, building materials, agrochemicals, genetically modified foods or plastic packaging.

Sourcing pastured and free-range animal protein

This will ensure a beneficial nutrient ratio which includes the protective fatty acid CLA (conjugated linoleic acid). When you include bone broths and the fats of pastured animals the quantity of protein required can be minimised as glycine-rich broths are both protective and protein 'sparing'. Collagen from bone broth aids in the healing of the digestive tract and can assist in reducing food reactivity.

Including good amount of quality fats and oils will support brain function and detoxification pathway

Consuming quality fats helps to stimulate

bile production and subsequently the elimination of toxins through the bowel. For cooking purposes choose pastured animal fats, duck or goose fat or coconut oil and of course ghee. For cold dishes, pesto, dips and dressings use cold pressed virgin olive oil, fresh avocado and essential fatty acid-rich cold, pressed oils such as Inchi oil or nut and seed oils. Avoid all industrially extracted seed and vegetable oils, soybean or rice bran oil, commercial fried foods and margarines which are prone to oxidation and will only serve to increase oxidative stress in the body.

Choose safe, sustainable seafoods

Choose fresh, wild, small, oily fish as a source of anti-inflammatory omega 3s. Download the 'Smart Seafood Buying Guide' from the NRDC web site and avoid fish species which are prone to mercury bioaccumulation.

Antioxidant-rich foods will help to protect you on a cellular level from the ravages of free radical oxidative stress

The following foods are excellent sources of antioxidants.

- Vitamin A: Cod liver oil, organic pastured liver/ Pâté, wild fish eggs
- Vitamin C and carotenoids: fermented and fresh, raw, colourful vegetables and wild berries
- CoQ10: pastured, organic, heart meat is a rich source of this antioxidant and energy-supportive element.
- Selenium: Brazil nuts, sustainable, 'smart' seafoods
- Phytonutrients: fresh and organic dried herbs and spices including oregano (great for candida/ yeast infections), rosemary (helpful in detoxifying excess estrogen and supporting memory function), dill, fennel, anise and caraway seeds to support digestion and microbial balance. Green tea polyphenols.

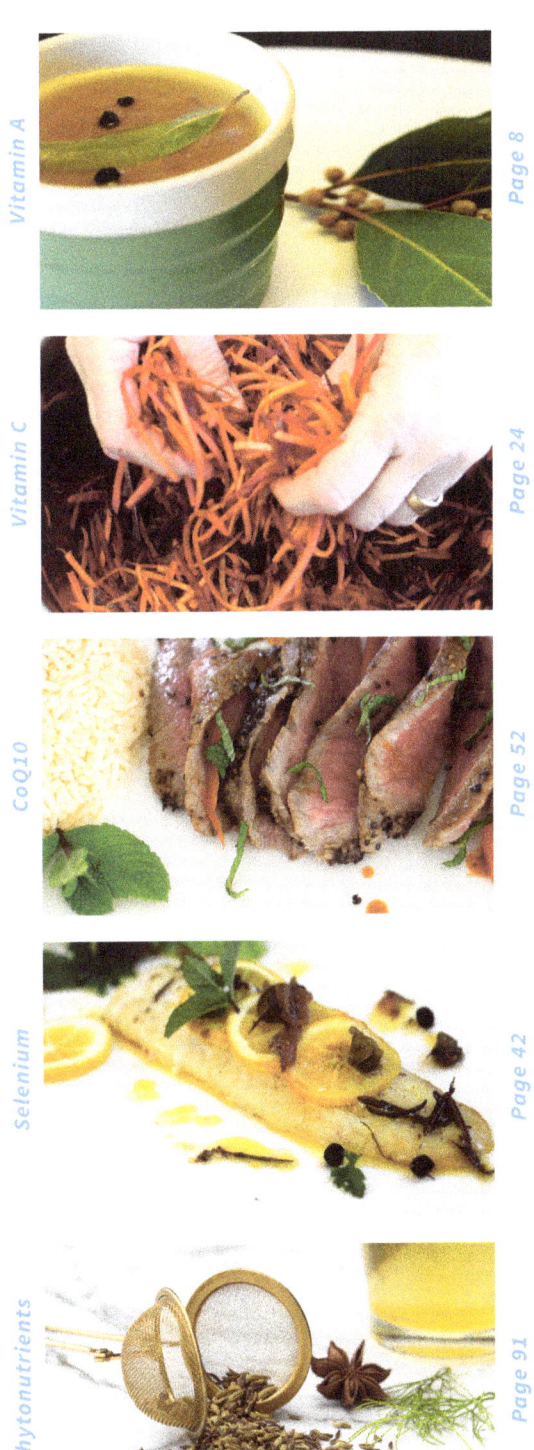

xxi

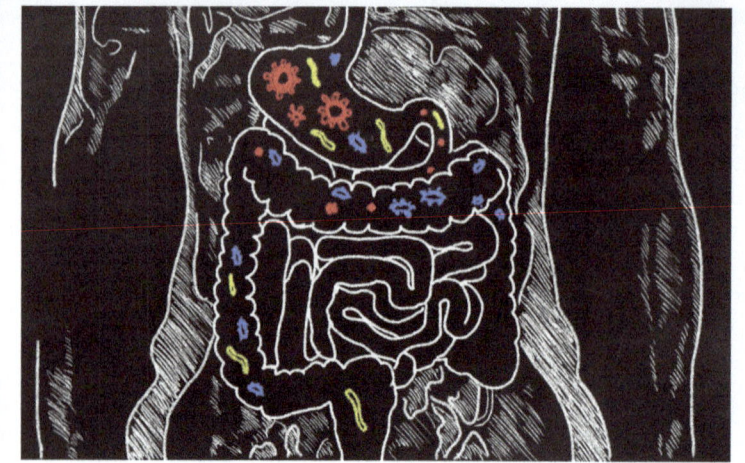

Restoring a healthy microbial balance in the digestive tract will in turn reduce your uptake of heavy metals.

Mercury toxic people are commonly depleted in minerals, particularly magnesium and zinc

Optimising your mineral status will aid in the displacement of heavy metals as you chelate them out of the body. Choose from as broad a range of plant foods, herbs, spices and protein-rich foods as possible. Most people will need to supplement these minerals in the short term whilst addressing their heavy metals and/or undertaking a restrictive diet.

Foods and nutrients which support kidney function

One of the main pathways of elimination for chelated mercury is via the kidneys. Ginger and parsley are excellent low thiol options which feature in many of our recipes.

Foods and nutrients which support liver function

The liver similarly is responsible for the detoxification of mercury and as such is commonly adversely impacted by heavy metals. Milk thistle taken as tea or supplement can be very effective.

Manage fungal infections naturally

It's not uncommon to find fungal infections such as Candida Albicans in those with mercury toxicity as immune function is commonly suppressed. I have found that a better approach is to keep candida in check rather than try to eliminate it entirely. Fresh oregano and clove bud may be helpful as are the herbs Horopito and Pau D'arco. Be cautious of natural remedies oregano oil and grapefruit seed extract (GSE) as these have been found to damage the beneficial microbes along with pathogenic species.

Hemp Protein

Hemp seeds / protein is not only an excellent source of essential fatty acids it will also boost protein levels in support of a reduced animal protein intake.

Optimising your mineral status will aid in the displacement of heavy metals as you chelate them out of the body.

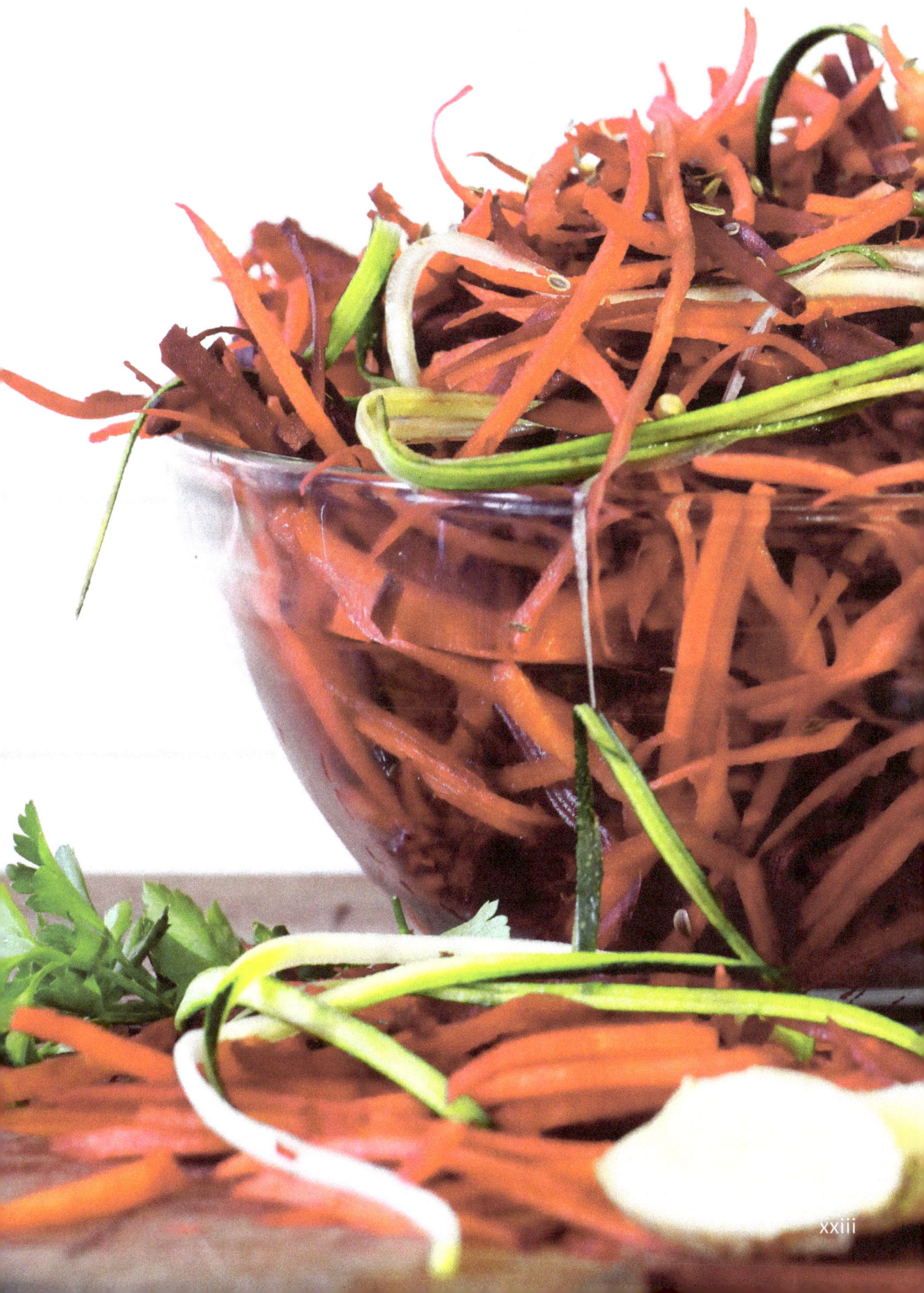

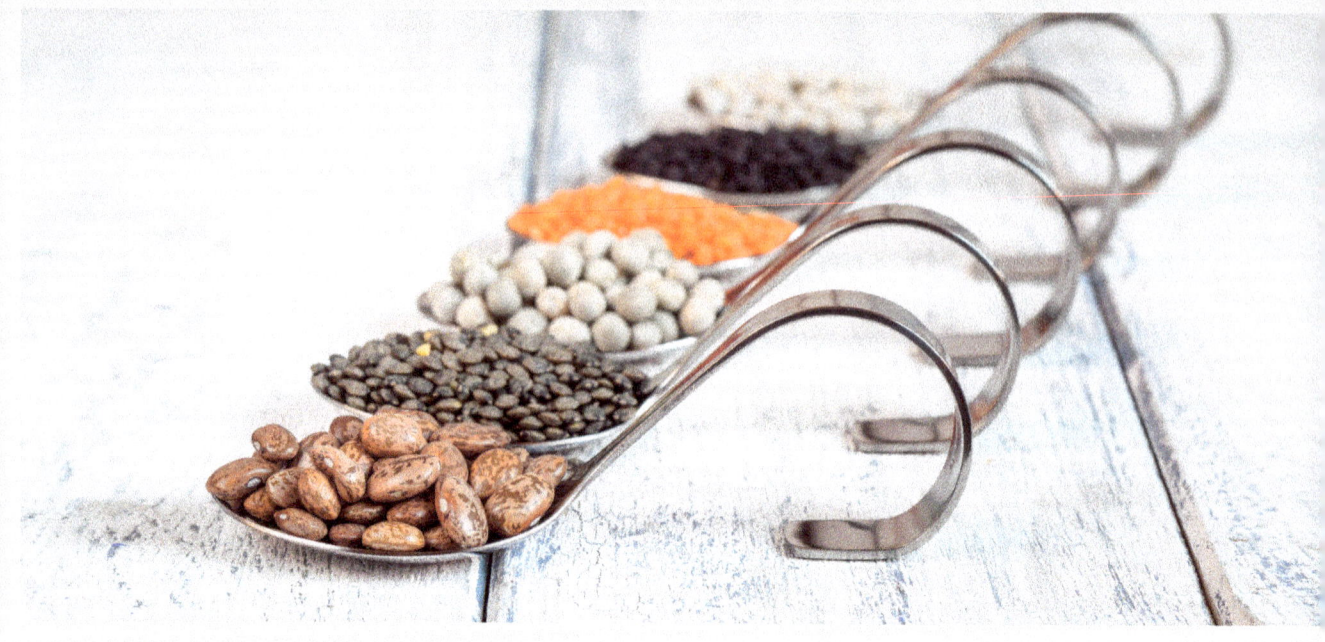

Grains, legumes, nuts and seeds

Grains

Should we include grains? Or avoid them?

We've known for some time now that refining and processing grains to remove their outer layers reduces their nutrient content. It is for this reason that we are told that whole grains are the healthier option. Proponents of the Paleo (Paleolithic) movement argue however that the consumption of grains is relatively new to man and is linked to modern, inflammatory diseases. We are told that grains together with legumes for this reason should be avoided.

This premise ignores the early 20th century work of Dr Weston A. Price who found that many traditional groups in the far reaches of the preindustrial, globe had a common set of rules related to the consumption of grains. Thanks to scientific methods we can now begin to understand more fully the 'why' of the food preparation practices that the good doctor observed in his travels.[1] This is because grains contain compounds which are designed to protect them in nature from sprouting prematurely. These anti-nutrients are natures' armor and include **enzyme inhibitors**, **indigestible sugars**, **phytic acid** and complex protein structures including **gluten**. Modern methods of food processing ignore these compounds to our detriment, resulting in indigestion, malabsorption, mineral deficiencies and neurological disturbances.

Traditional peoples knew that mimicking nature resulted in the dismantling of these digestive disrupters. When we soak, sprout and sour our grains the seed is triggered to switch from protective mode to growth mode, unlocking its energy reserves for nourishment.[2]

Gluten

Every second person seems to be intolerant! Or is there something else at play?

For a percentage of us with a genetic predisposition, gluten-containing grains are a 'no go'. For many more of us however processed grains can cause considerable pain despite a negative celiac test result.

The widespread use of the broad-spectrum herbicide Roundup (glyphosate) on grain and food crops is raising suspicion as the culprit behind a surge in inflammatory conditions. Senior research scientist Dr. Stephanie Seneff presents the mechanisms by which Roundup has the potential to cause considerable harm to both our internal and external environments. Glyphosate disrupts the shikimate pathway in microbes therefore disturbing the delicate balance in both our gut and our soil microbiota. Could this explain the increased rates of non-celiac digestive inflammation and food intolerances?

As more and more research into our microbial population emerges the link becomes clear.[3]

If you know that you are not celiac and your digestive system is in good order then by all means include organic, spray-free, gluten and non-gluten grains in your low-thiol protocol. Do however ensure that you

a Choose organic, spray free grains, and

b You prepare them appropriately by soaking, souring, sprouting and cooking them according to the wise traditions of our forefathers.[4]

You are what you assimilate

Preparing your grains, nuts, seeds and legumes for optimal digestion and assimilation:

Equipment

A good quality dehydrator recommended, particularly for families wishing to prepare their own activated nuts, grains and surplus produce at home. I use Excalibur brand dehydrator to make yogurt also as the shelves can be removed leaving room for large jars.

Pure filtered water: chlorinate and fluoridated water will damage naturally occurring microbes and enzymes in your food and your gut. There are a number of efficient filtration systems available. The most important question to ask is does it remove fluoride as well as chlorine.

A food processor for your grains. I like Vitamix or Thermomix. The Vitamix 'dry bowl' is great for grinding dry grains into flour or meal.

Nuts and Seeds

You may be familiar with the term 'activated' when it comes to nuts and seeds. Have you wondered if it is worth the bother or the expense of purchasing them already activated? Nuts and seeds like grains contain anti-nutrients which when ignored can lead to symptoms of digestive irritability, bloating and altered bowel function. Mercury can dismantle digestive enzymes further compounding digestive disorders. In a nut shell, we need all the nutrient help we can get and a simple soaking of your nuts and seeds is an excellent place to begin.

---

1 Weston A. Price, DDS 2011 Nutrition and Physical Degeneration 8th edition. Price-Pottenger Nutrition Foundation
2 Fallon S., Enig M. 2000 Be kind to your grains.... And Your Grains will be kind to you The Weston A. Price Foundation.
3 Samsel A., Seneff S. 2013 Glyphosate, pathways to modern diseases II: Celiac sprue and gluten intolerance J of Interdisciplinary Toxicology.
4 Fallon S. Enig M., 2001 Nourishing Traditions, The Cookbook that Challenges Politically Correct Nutrition and the Diet Dictocrats, Revised 2nd edition. New Trend Publishing.

Activating nuts and seeds

If you do not own a dehydrator you can still activate your nuts and seeds. They will need to be eaten within a few hours of activation or refrigerated for up to 24 hours. Once dehydrated however they can be stored in an airtight container in a cool place for many weeks provided they are crispy dry. Very small seeds such as poppy or sesame seeds need not be activated. Flax and chia seeds are best soaked for an hour or so and then eaten.

1. Place a good quantity of nuts into a non-metallic bowl. Allow room at the top for them to expand by around one third
2. Cover with warm, pure water and add 1 Tbs of salt for every 2L of water
3. Stir the salt into the water. Cover loosely with a tea towel and place in a warm area
4. Leave for 4 - 6 hours, drain and transfer to the dehydrator
5. Dry at around 45°C for around 24 - 36 hours depending on the size of the nut or seed. Most important is that they are crispy dry to avoid mold growth during storage

Once you've tasted crispy, activated nuts and seeds you can never go back to the raw, hard, dry version!

Grains

Whole, organically grown grains are delicious when soaked, sprouted or soured.

Traditional groups prepared grains for their flat breads, soups, stews and porridge by soaking their grains or freshly ground gruel in pure water. They would often add a 'starter' such as raw whey or milk as a source of beneficial microbes. These bugs are effectively pre-digesting the otherwise disruptive compounds enabling easier assimilation of nutrients in our digestive tracts.

Whole grains for use in bread, flat bread, porridge, stew or soup.

1. Place whole grains in a non-metallic bowl. Cover with pure, filtered warm water and a splash of 'acidic' liquid such as lemon juice, whey (not permitted in low thiol diet) or kombucha
2. Rinse the grains under running, filtered water every 8 hours or so and top up the lemon juice or kombucha.
3. Soak whole grains for 24 - 36 hours, rinsing regularly
4. Drain and add to soups or stew or simmer to make a porridge. To make flat bread or sourdough grind the grains in a good quality food processor together with a 'starter' such as kombucha and allow the batter to prove in a warm place for around 4 hours before baking or frying
5. Dehydrate grains which will be stored, ground into flour or used in cookies and granola. Dry at 45°C for around 24 hours or until completely dry
6. Serve your grains with good quality fats such as ghee or coconut yogurt. Use raw cream or butter once you are including thiols again. These fats enable the uptake of minerals and nutrients from your grains

Legumes

The legume family includes lentils, dried beans, peas and peanuts. Whether they are soaked, soured or sprouted legumes remain on the 'no' list of the low thiol diet. When returning these valuable, nutrient and fiber-rich foods to your diet however the following rules will ensure that you extract all of their available nutrition.

For those with digestive disturbances even well-prepared legumes can cause symptoms of bloating and discomfort. It's for this reason that we remove them from healing protocols such as the GAPS diet (Gut and Psychology Syndrome) and

FODMAPS diet (Fermentable Oligo-, Di-, Mono-saccharides and Polyols). We can return correctly prepared legumes to the diet beginning with red and brown lentils followed by white beans and then on to coloured beans

Soy beans should never be consumed unfermented as they contain thyroid blocking compounds, vitamin B12 analogues which block B12 absorption and protein-breaking enzyme inhibitors.

1. Rinse the dried beans or lentils in large bowl. Pour off any floating or discoloured legumes
2. Cover the legumes with warm, filtered water with a pinch of bicarb soda added. Leave at room temperature
3. Lentils, split peas and white beans (Haricot) require a shorter time from 2 - 4 hours. Whilst other beans (Adzuki, Cannellini, Red Kidney, Black, Lima, whole peas, Chickpeas) require longer, an overnight soak is ideal
4. Rinse the legumes under running water
5. Simmer the legumes in plenty of pure water without salt. Adding a 4 - 6 inch piece of kombu to the cooking water will further reduce any flatulence effects
6. Drain and serve with good amounts of quality fats and or bone broth
7. Adding fermented vegetables or an acid dressing will further aid in digestibility of your legumes

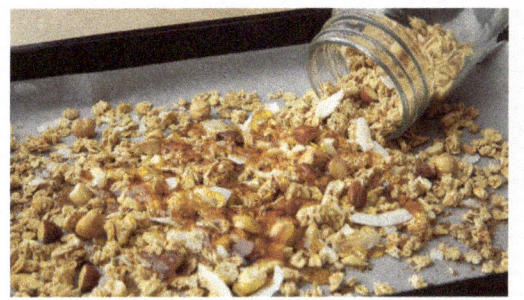

Page 5

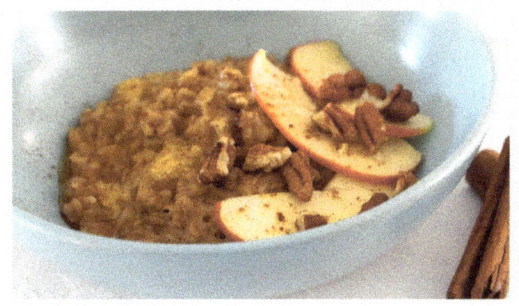

Page 11

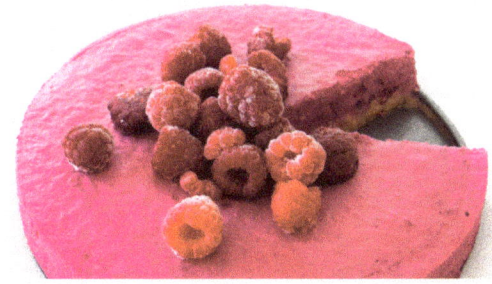

Page 69

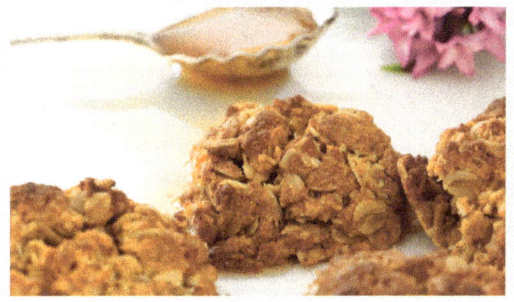

Page 77

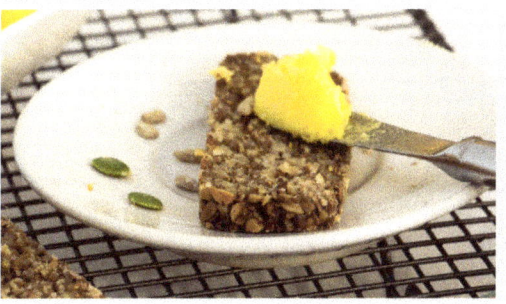

Page 84

Key

 Gluten Free

 Nut Free

 Dairy Free

Items marked dairy free may contain ghee which is commonly well tolerated. For those who do not tolerate ghee substitute cold-pressed, virgin olive, walnut or hazelnut oil for cold, raw dishes & substitute organic, pastured animal dripping, duck or goose fat for cooking purposes.

 Vegetarian

Items marked vegetarian may include ghee. Substitute animal fats with ghee or plant oils

 Sugar Free

Items marked sugar free may contain natural sweeteners such as maple syrup or honey. Where sugar in included we've opted for nutrient-rich forms such as coconut, palm or rapadura sugar. Ultimately sugar is sugar & should be avoided if you have health concerns such as obesity, diabetes, cardiovascular & other metabolic disorders.

Completion Time
The time required to prepare & serve the final dish.

Prep Time
Includes the time required for the preparation of of ingredients including pre-soaking, sprouting or fermenting.

Baking Conversion Charts

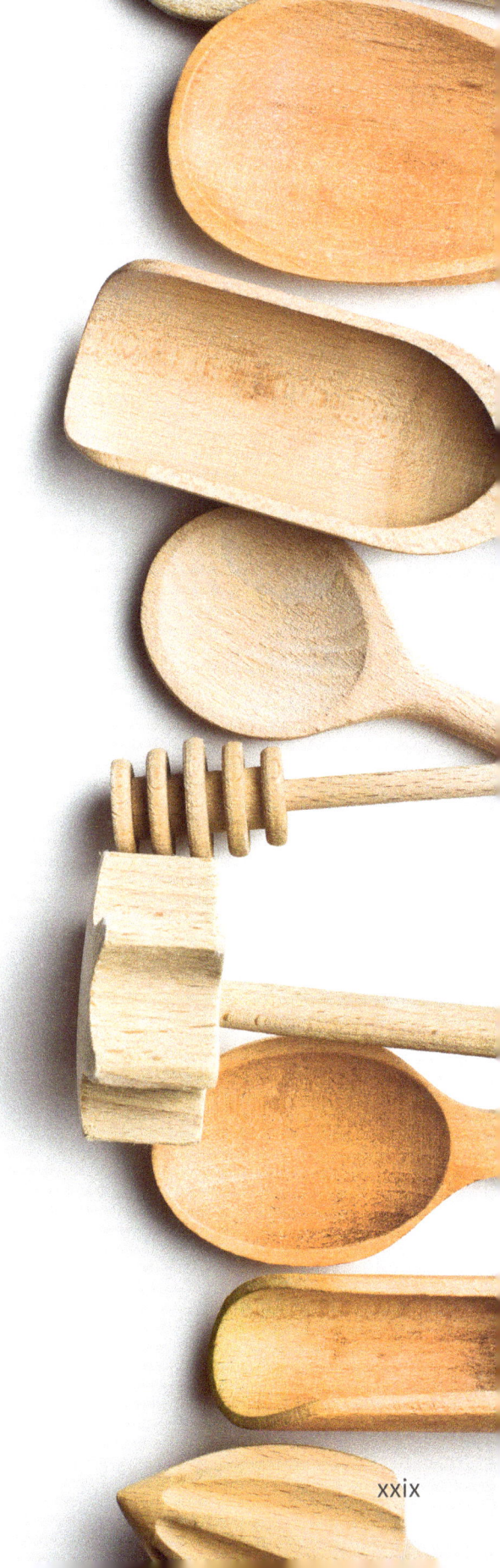

Spoon Cups	Liquid ml
1/4 tsp	1.25 ml
1/2 tsp	2.5 ml
1 tsp	5 ml
1 Tbs	15 ml
1/4 cup	60 ml
1/3 cup	80 ml
1/2 cup	125 ml
1 cup	250 ml

Dry measurements

1 Tbs	1/2 oz.	14 g
1/4 cup	2 oz.	56.7 g
1/3 cup	2.6 oz.	75.4 g
1/2 cup	4 oz.	113.4 g
3/4 cup	6 oz.	170 g
1 cup	8 oz.	227 g
2 cups	16 oz.	454 g

Volume Liquids

2 Tbs	1 fl. oz.	30 ml
1/4 cup	2 fl. oz.	60 ml
1/2 cup	4 fl. oz.	125 ml
1 cup	8 fl. oz.	250 ml
1.5 cups	12 fl. oz.	375 ml
2 cups	16 fl. oz. / 1 pint	500 ml
4 cups	32 fl. oz. / 1 quart	1000 ml / 1 l

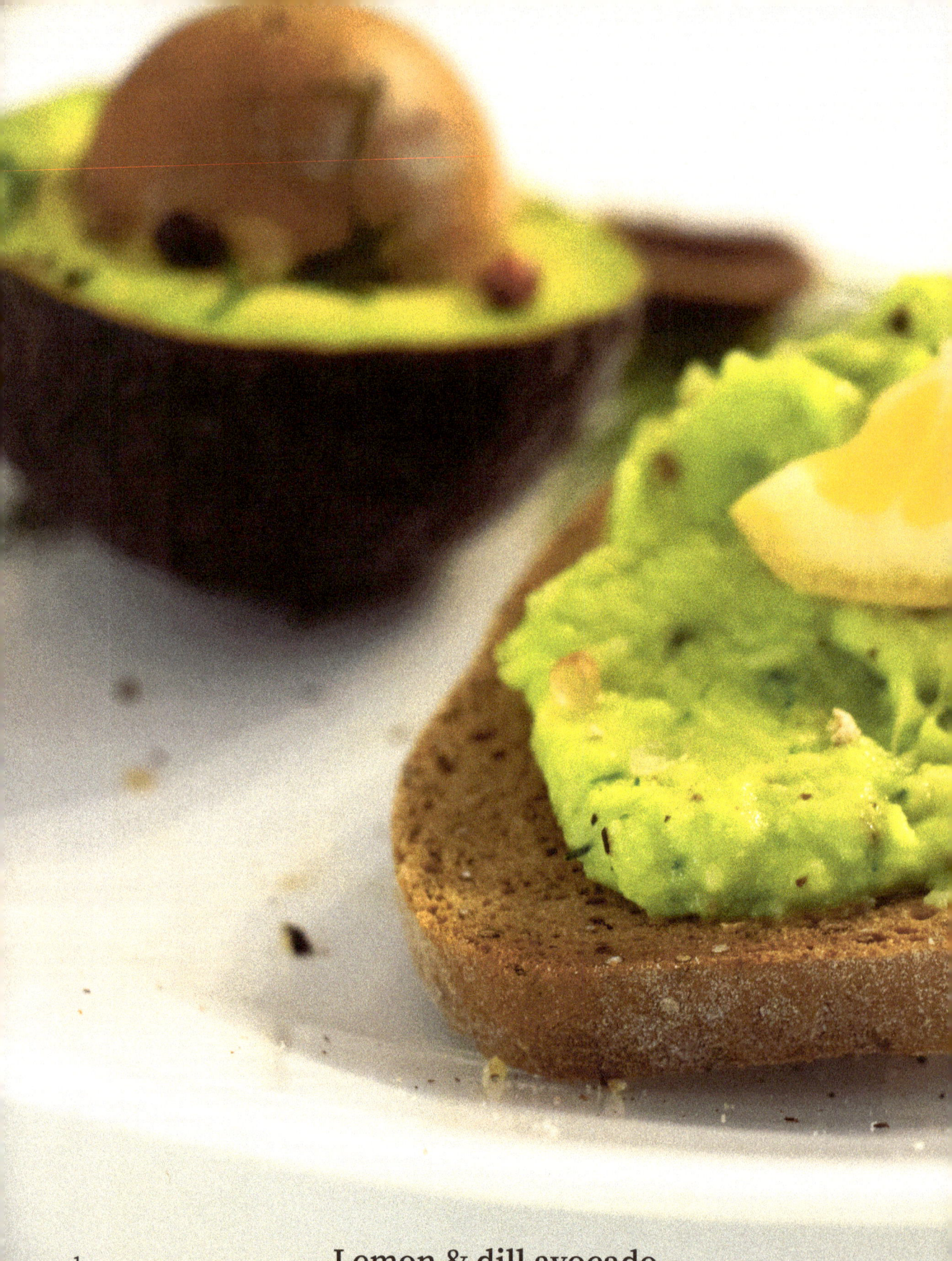

Lemon & dill avocado p3

RISE & SHINE
the morning's fine

Lemon & dill avocado	3	Mushrooms with basil	9
Avocado with bacon & parsley	3	Spiced apple with ginger & orange zest	10
Honey nut granola	5	Creamy spiced porridge	11
Banana pancakes	6	Chai tea chia pudding	12
Mushroom pâté	7		
Organic turkey, duck or chicken liver pâté	8		

Lemon & dill avocado

COMPLETION TIME: 5 min

LEVEL: Easy

PREP: 1 min

YIELD: 2 servings

Ingredients

1 large ripe avocado halved

1 tsp dill finely chopped

1 tsp mint leaves finely chopped

1 Tbs fresh lemon or lime juice

1 Tbs hazelnut or walnut oil*

salt and pepper to season

*NOTE: These oils are commonly available from good delis and health stores in dark glass or tins. If not available use cold pressed organic Virgin Olive Oil.

Method

1. Roughly mash the avocado and place into a bowl with chopped dill, mint, salt and pepper and the lemon or lime juice
2. Mix to combine and serve drizzled with oil
3. Serve on a slice or two of toasted Olive and Oregano Seed Loaf

Avocado with bacon & parsley

Ingredients

1 large ripe avocado halved

2 Tbs fresh parsley finely chopped

4 or more fresh Swiss Brown mushrooms diced or sliced

1 large rasher of free-range, nitrate-free bacon chopped

1 Tbs organic ghee

salt and pepper to season

Method

1. In a large fry pan sauté the bacon and mushrooms in ghee until tender
2. Add the parsley and continue to sauté
3. Serve the mushrooms over the halved avocado and top with slices of lemon, salt and pepper

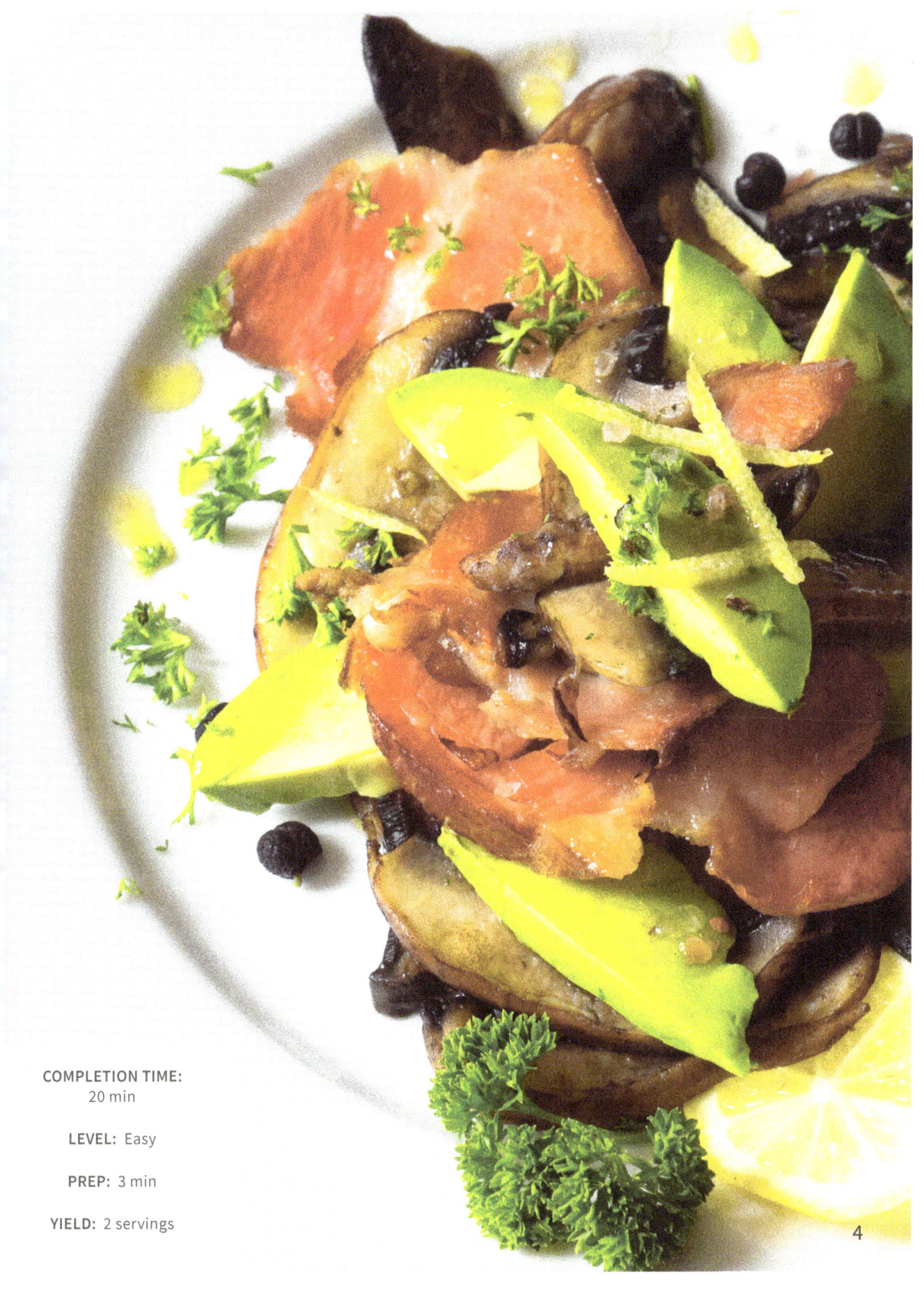

COMPLETION TIME:
20 min

LEVEL: Easy

PREP: 3 min

YIELD: 2 servings

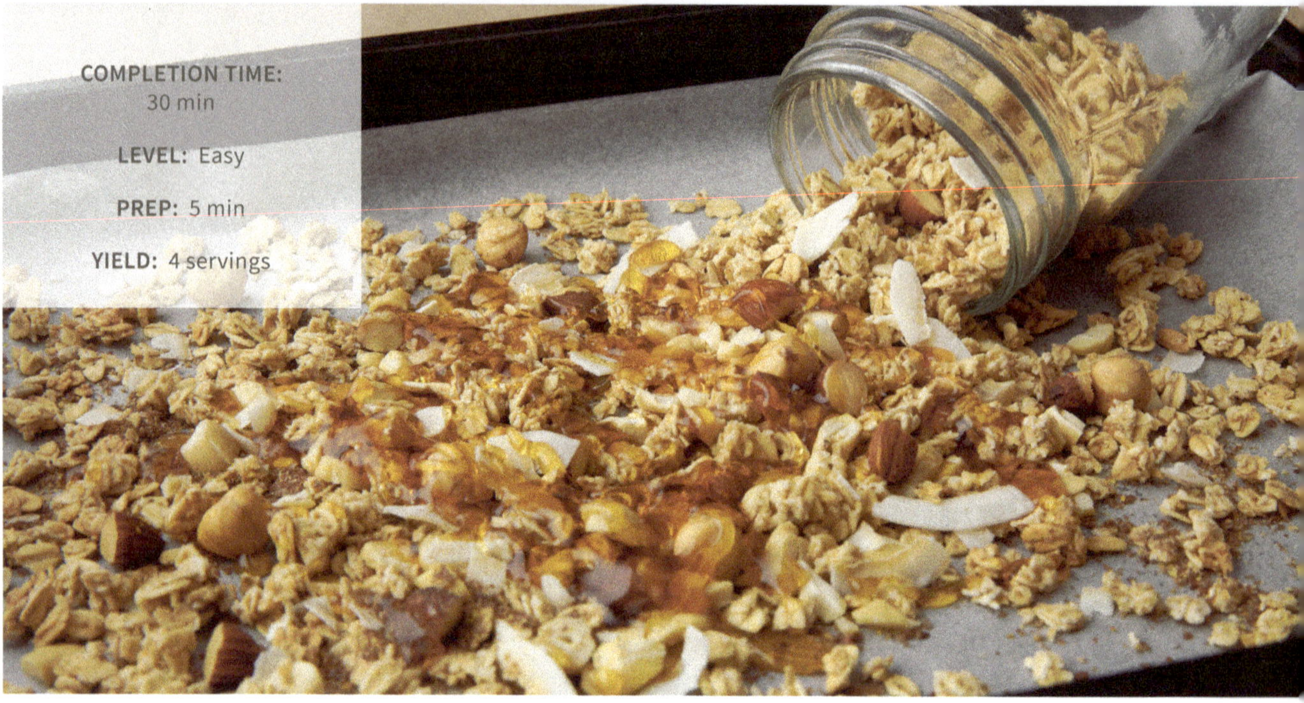

COMPLETION TIME: 30 min

LEVEL: Easy

PREP: 5 min

YIELD: 4 servings

Honey nut granola

Gluten Free

Vegetarian

Dairy Free

Ingredients

2 1/2 cups soaked* organic rolled oats

1/2 cup shredded coconut

1/2 cup activated* brazil nuts chopped

1/4 cup activated* hazelnuts chopped

3 Tbs ghee

3 Tbs *Nut butter* (p98)

1 Tbs rapadura or coconut sugar

2 tsp raw honey

2 Tbs psyllium husk

Option: Any choice of nut in the same quantity may be substituted for the brazil nuts and hazelnuts.

Method

1. Preheat oven to 180°C or 350°F
2. Combine the ghee, nut butter, Rapadura sugar and honey in a saucepan over a low heat to melt
3. Remove the saucepan from the heat
4. Add to dry ingredients and mix well
5. Spread mixture onto the lined baking tray
6. Toast in the oven for 10 minutes or until golden, mixing a couple of times to prevent burning
7. Allow cooling, transfer to an airtight container and refrigerate
8. Serve with your choice of non-dairy milk

*For more information about why it is important to soak and dry oats and activate nuts, see page xxiv

Banana pancakes

Gluten Free　Nut Free　Vegetarian　Sugar Free

Heavy metal toxicity often causes digestive weakness as a result of reduced digestive enzymes. Lightly fermenting the batter using a live culture or starter aids in the break down of anti-nutrients found in grains.

Ingredients

2 ripe bananas mashed

1 cup organic rice flour (can be ground in a Thermomix or Vitamix dry bowl)

1 cup organic oat flour (can be ground in a Thermomix or Vitamix dry bowl)

1 tsp gluten free, aluminium-free baking powder

1/2 tsp Himalayan salt

2 tsp Sweet Spice Blend

1 cup (less 2 Tbs) organic coconut milk (nut-free option) or activated almond milk

2 tsp honey

1 Tbs melted coconut oil

1 tsp vanilla extract (optional)

1 Tbs ghee for greasing pan

2 Tbs *Kombucha (p93)* or water kefir or plain coconut yogurt to use as a starter

Method

1. In a food processor blend the milk, honey, vanilla, starter and coconut oil, add mashed bananas and blend further to a smooth consistency
2. Beat in rice flour, oat flour, baking powder, salt and spice blend with a wooden spoon
3. Allow the batter to sit in a warm place covered with a clean cloth for around 4 - 6 hours or overnight
4. Place 1/4 cup of mixture into a hot greased pan and cook lightly on both sides for a couple of minutes
5. Serve warm or cold topped with *Jillaine's raw honey drizzle* (p68) or *Whipped creamy coconut* (p68) and slices of banana

Vegan option: Replace butter with coconut oil.

Grain-free option: Banana flour and tapioca starch can also be used and will provide resistant starch which is great for feeding your gut microbes.

COMPLETION TIME: 40 min

LEVEL: Moderate

PREP: 6-8 hours

YIELD: 4 servings
Makes 8 - 10 pancakes

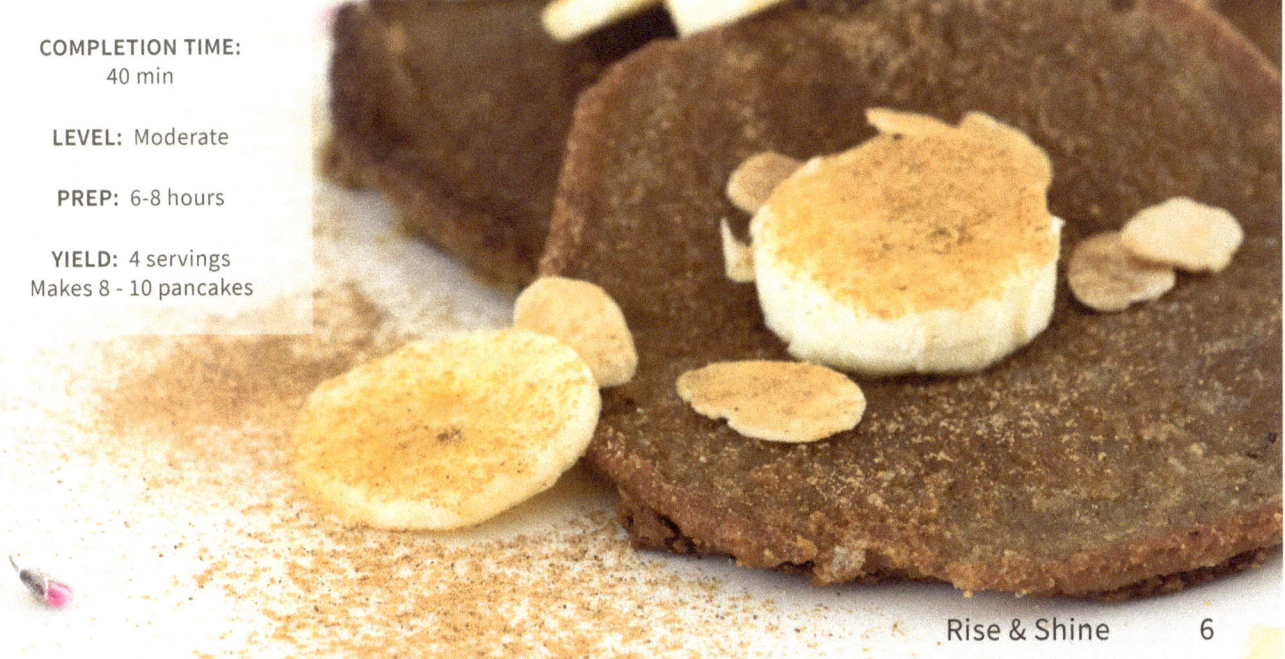

Rise & Shine

Mushroom pâté

Gluten Free | Vegetarian | Dairy Free | Sugar Free

Certain mushroom varieties have medicinal properties. They support immune function and have antiviral and antibacterial properties. Varieties include Shiitaki, Chaga, Maitake Lion's Mane, Cordyceps, Reishi, Turkey tail all of which can be purchased in dried form and rehydrated for cooking together with local culinary mushrooms.

Ingredients

1/4 cup of dried mushrooms. Use Porcini or French forest mix or varieties listed above

1/4 cup pure water

1 cup sliced Swiss brown mushrooms

1/2 cup chopped parsley

1 tsp thyme

1/4 tsp freshly shaved nutmeg

1/2 tsp gluten-free asafoetida

1 Tbs ghee or duck fat

1-2 Tbs cold-pressed olive oil

salt and pepper to season

cashew *Nut butter* *(p98)*

the juice of half a lemon

Method

1. Soak the dried mushrooms in water for a few hours
2. Heat the duck fat or ghee in a medium fry pan
3. Sauté the fresh mushrooms together with the soaked mushrooms and the soaking liquid until the liquid is reduced
4. Add the herbs and spice and continue sautéing until fragrant and the mushrooms are softened
5. Set aside to cool
6. In a good food processor blend the mushroom mixture, nut butter and lemon juice until smooth
7. Add olive oil if needed to achieve a smooth consistency
8. Spoon into ramekins and top with a slice of fried mushroom and a sprig of parsley and a drizzle of olive oil
9. Refrigerate until firm and serve with *Seed crackers* *(p85)*

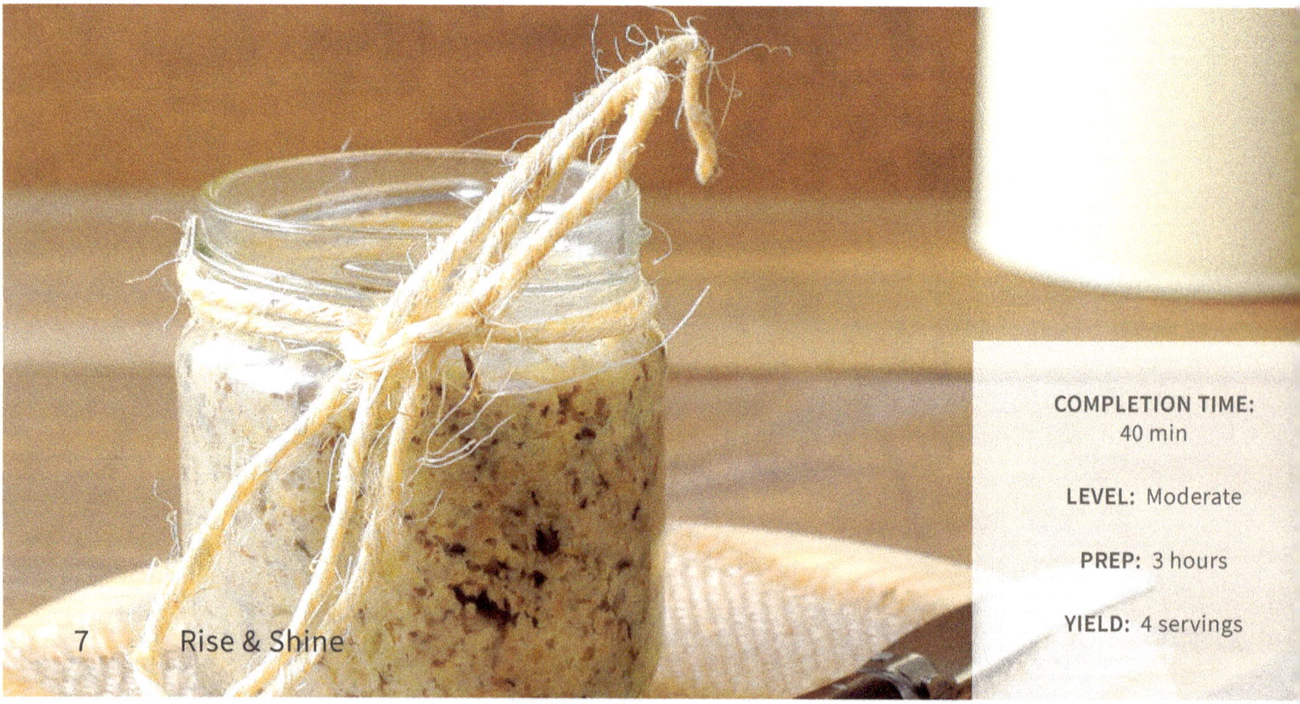

COMPLETION TIME: 40 min

LEVEL: Moderate

PREP: 3 hours

YIELD: 4 servings

Organic turkey, duck or chicken liver pâté

Contrary to popular opinion, liver does not accumulate but rather processes toxin for removal from the body. Good quality organic liver from free range animals is a superior source of nutrients and is considered a 'sacred' food by traditional groups. Not surprising considering its nutrient content- in particular those nutrients which support detoxification.

Ingredients

500g raw organic livers

2 tsp fresh or dried thyme

1-2 rashers of nitrate and sugar-free bacon roughly chopped

2 Tbs of chopped parsley

1/2 tsp gluten-free Asafoetida powder (garlic replacer)

cracked pepper and sea or Himalayan salt to taste

200g ghee or use duck or goose fat if you are dairy free

sufficient bone broth reduction to get the mixture running smoothly in the food processor

Method

1. Heat ghee or duck fat in a heavy skillet. Add 2 Tbs of broth, chopped bacon and thyme and fry gently until tender, stirring occasionally. Set aside in a large bowl

2. Turn up the heat a little, add more fat and add chicken, duck or turkey livers- giving them space in the pan to brown rather than broil. Add parsley pepper and salt to taste. Turn the livers after a couple of minutes and brown the other side

3. Make sure the livers are just brown on the outside and still pink on the inside. Remove from heat and allow to cool a little

4. Process all of the ingredients in a food processor with melted gelatinous bone broth Thermomix speed 6 until smooth or to your liking. Smooth or slightly lumpy, French style

5. Pour into ceramic bowls or glass jars and add some fried, fresh sage leaves on top. Melt some more ghee or duck fat and pour over the pâté. This seals the pâté and the sage has been used for many years to ward off insects

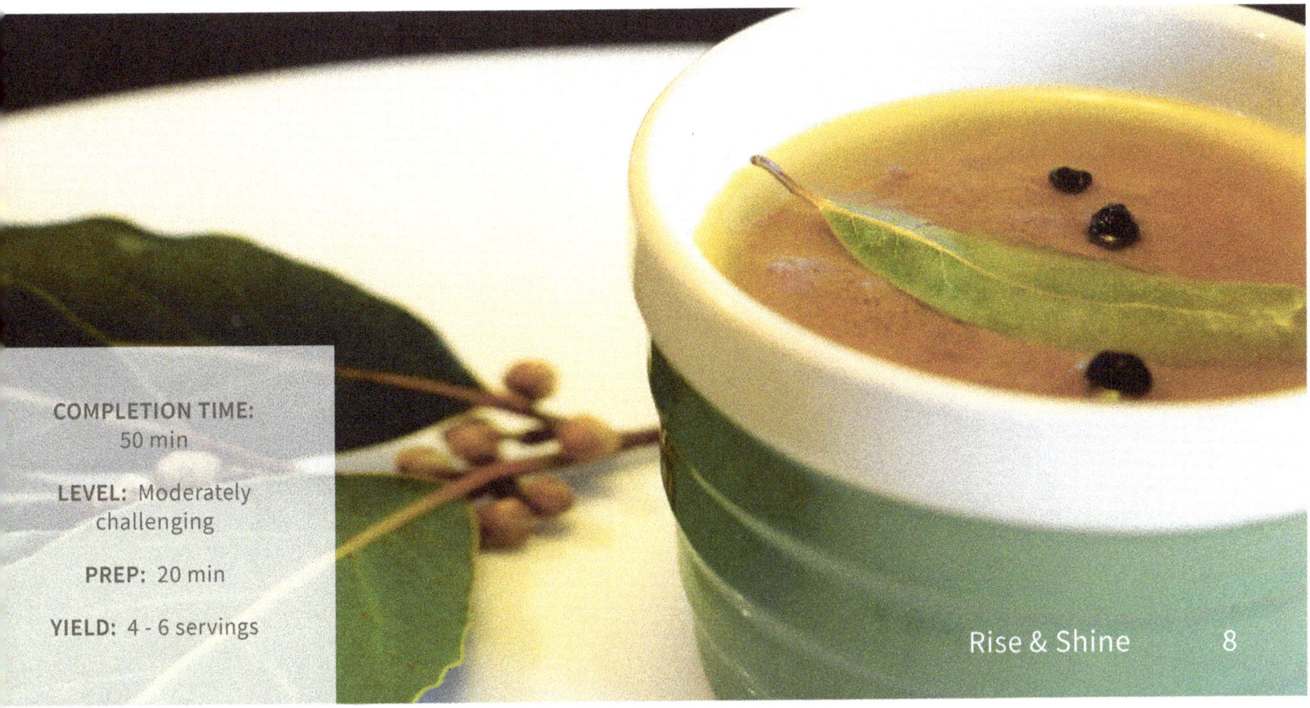

COMPLETION TIME: 50 min

LEVEL: Moderately challenging

PREP: 20 min

YIELD: 4 - 6 servings

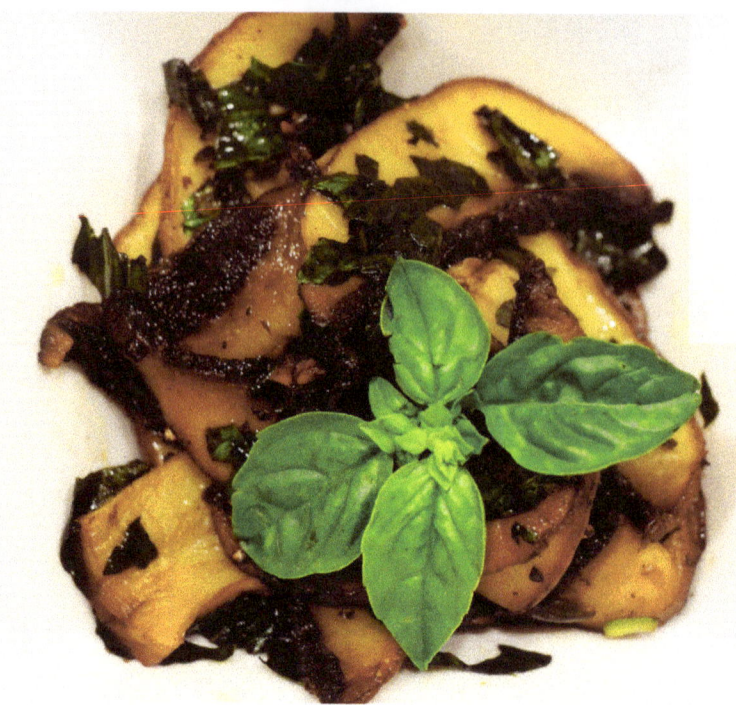

COMPLETION TIME: 20 min

LEVEL: Easy

PREP: 5 min

YIELD: 2 servings

Mushrooms with basil

Gluten Free   Nut Free   Vegetarian   Dairy Free   Sugar Free

Ingredients

1 cup sliced mushrooms of your choice

1/4 cup shredded basil leaves

1 Tbs organic ghee

2 Tbs chicken or vegetable *Stock* (p40)

Method

1. Sauté the sliced mushrooms in ghee and stock using a moderately hot frypan to soften the mushrooms and to release the flavour. Allow the stock to reduce to a sauce
2. Once slightly browned and softened remove from the heat
3. Toss with basil leaves, salt and pepper
4. Serve

Note: Most people who do not tolerate dairy do tolerate ghee as the proteins and lactose have been removed leaving just the oil portion.

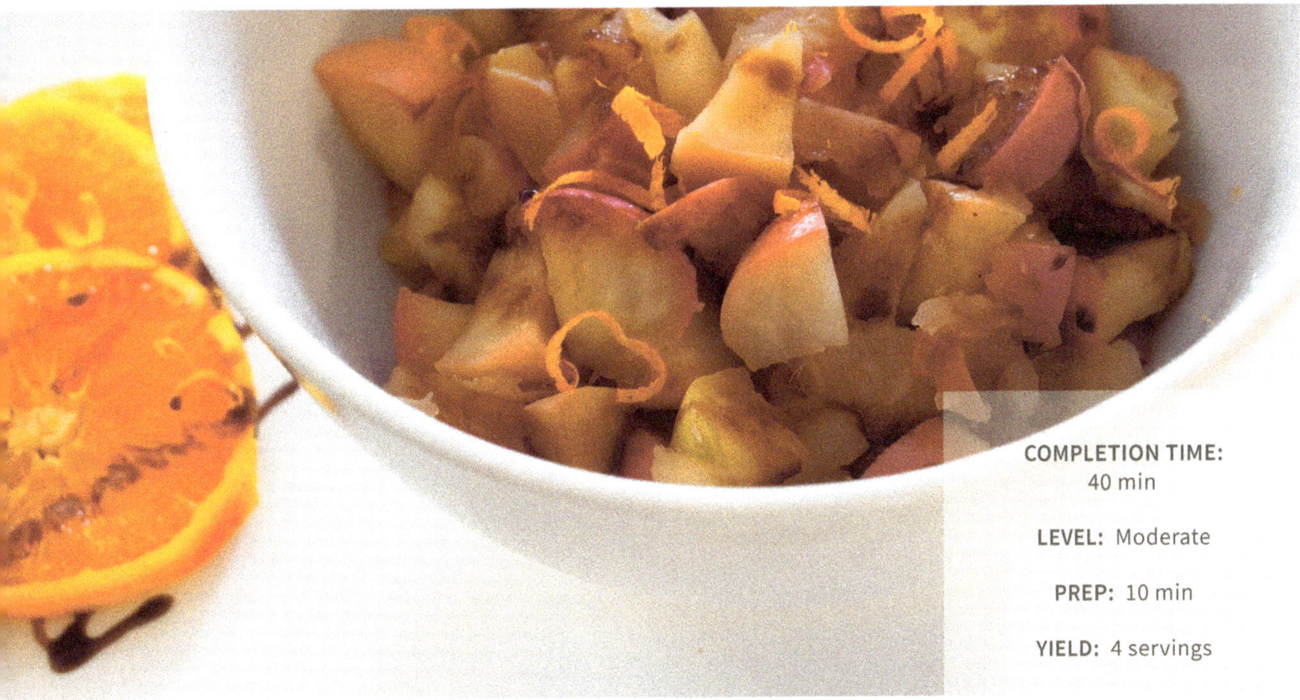

COMPLETION TIME: 40 min

LEVEL: Moderate

PREP: 10 min

YIELD: 4 servings

Spiced apple with ginger & orange zest

Gluten Free · Nut Free · Vegetarian · Dairy Free

Ingredients

1 1/2 kilos of granny smith, gravenstein or any other tart apple, peeled cored and diced

2 Tbs pure water

1 Tbs of rapadura or coconut sugar

1 Tbs of lemon juice

1 tsp grated fresh ginger

1 tsp of orange zest

1 tsp pomegranate molasses

Method

1. Place apples, sugar, ginger and water in a saucepan and heat until bubbling, reduce heat, cover with lid and gently simmer for 15 - 20 minutes
2. Add orange zest and a drizzle of Pomegranate Molasses. Serve hot or cold.

Spiced apple is delicious served on top of our *Creamy spiced porridge* (p11)

Rise & Shine

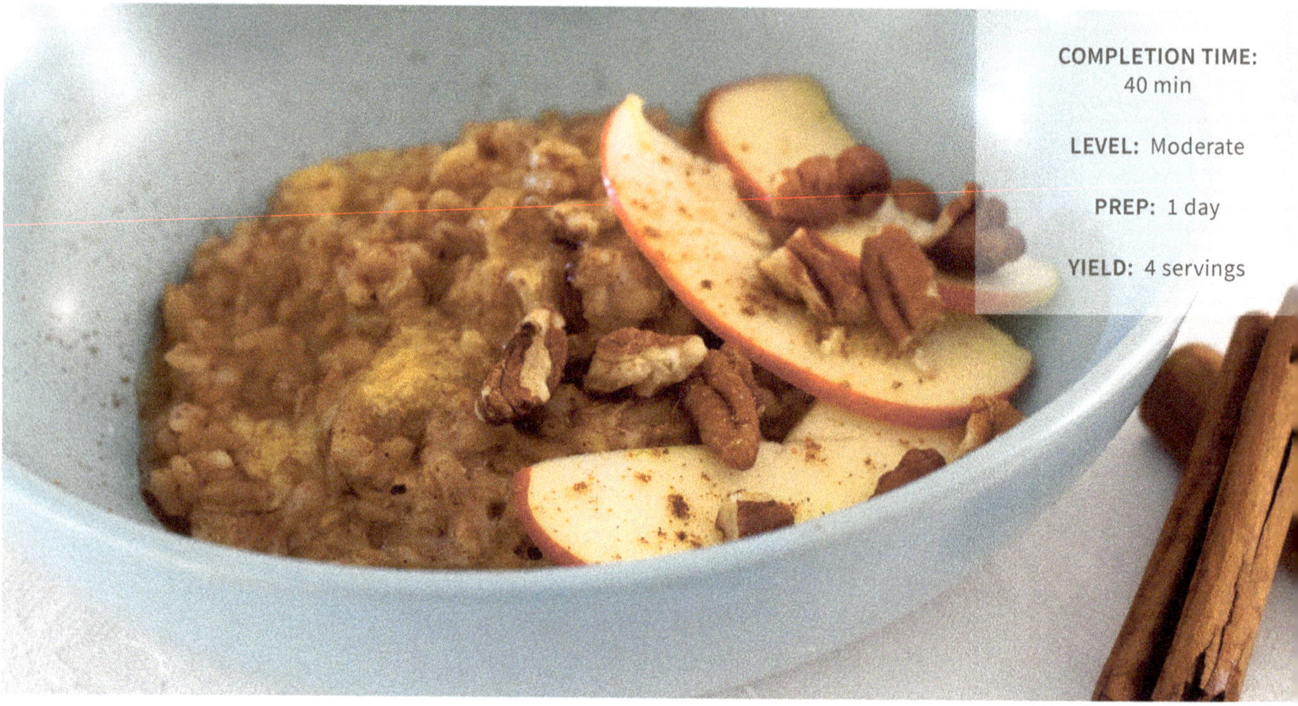

COMPLETION TIME: 40 min

LEVEL: Moderate

PREP: 1 day

YIELD: 4 servings

Creamy spiced porridge

 Gluten Free   Vegetarian   Dairy Free   Sugar Free

Ingredients

1 cup whole oat groats

1/2 cup millet

1/2 cup whole sorghum

1/4 cup red rice and/ or black rice

pure filtered water for soaking- enough to cover the grains

1 1/2 cups activated*, *Nut milk* (p95) or coconut milk

2 tsp of *Sweet spice blend* (p100)

pinch of Himalayan salt

1 apple grated

1/4 cup activated* pecan nuts chopped

1 - 2 tsp raw local honey or pure maple syrup

Method

1. Soak the grains in pure water for 24 hours*. Rinsing them once or twice during this time. Drain and rinse through a fine sieve
2. Mix the grains, almond milk, spice blend and salt in a saucepan over a medium heat and simmer for about 15 - 20 minutes
3. Add grated apple and pecan nuts and serve whilst hot topped with *Jillaine's raw honey drizzle* (p68)

Variation

Stewed apple, dates or apricots may be added when serving for extra variety. Top with a dollop of *Whipped creamy coconut* (p68)

NOTE: If you are Coeliac or gluten intolerant do check that the oats are processed or packaged in a gluten-free facility.
*For more information about why it is important to soak oats, grains and activate nuts, see page xxiv

Chai tea chia pudding

Gluten Free · Nut Free · Vegetarian · Dairy Free · Sugar Free

Ingredients

2 cups *Chai tea (p92)* made on your choice of activated* almond milk, coconut milk or rice milk (nut-free options)

1/2 cup chia seeds

5 drops pure vanilla extract

1/4 cup pure maple syrup or warmed raw honey

Method

1. Place all ingredients in blender and blend on high for about 2 minutes or until smooth
2. If you prefer a whole chia version, leave the chia seeds out, blend other ingredients first and then stir through the chia seeds
3. Pour mixture into a bowl or individual cups
4. Sprinkle with ground cinnamon
5. Refrigerate until chilled and firm
6. Serve with *Whipped creamy coconut (p68)*

*For more information about why it is important to activate nuts and seeds, see page xxiv

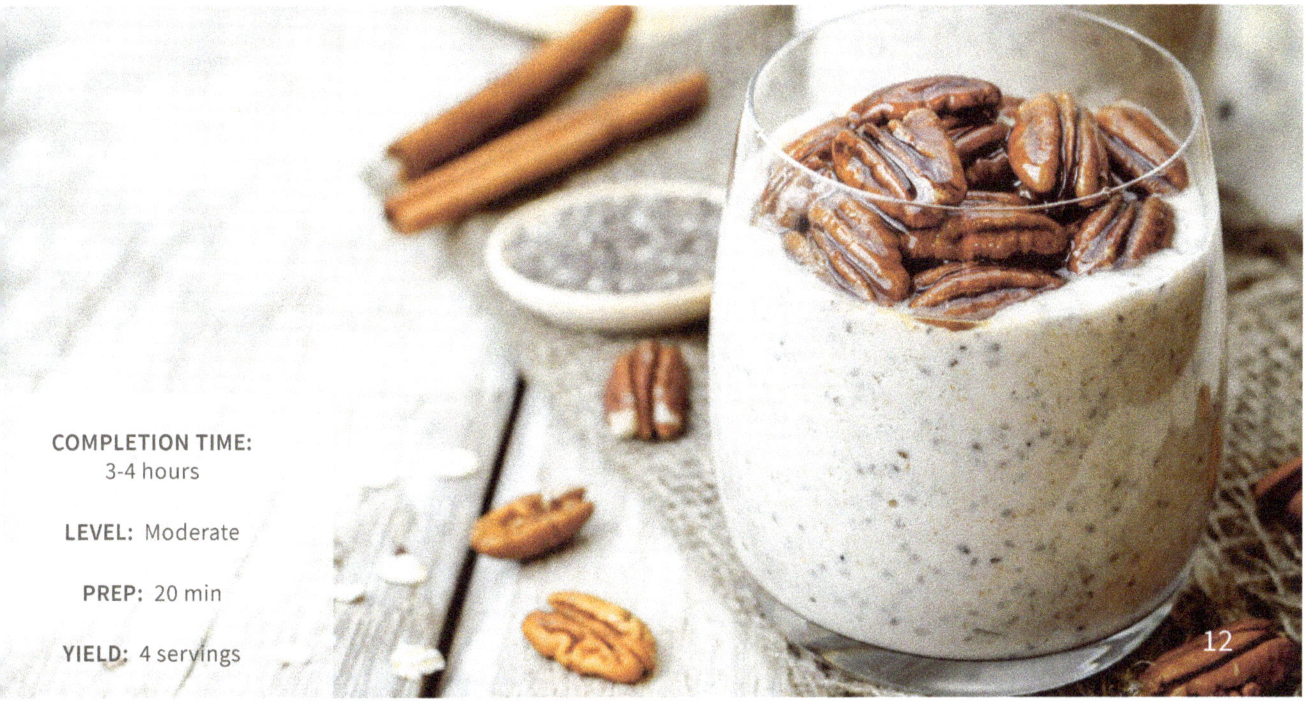

COMPLETION TIME: 3-4 hours

LEVEL: Moderate

PREP: 20 min

YIELD: 4 servings

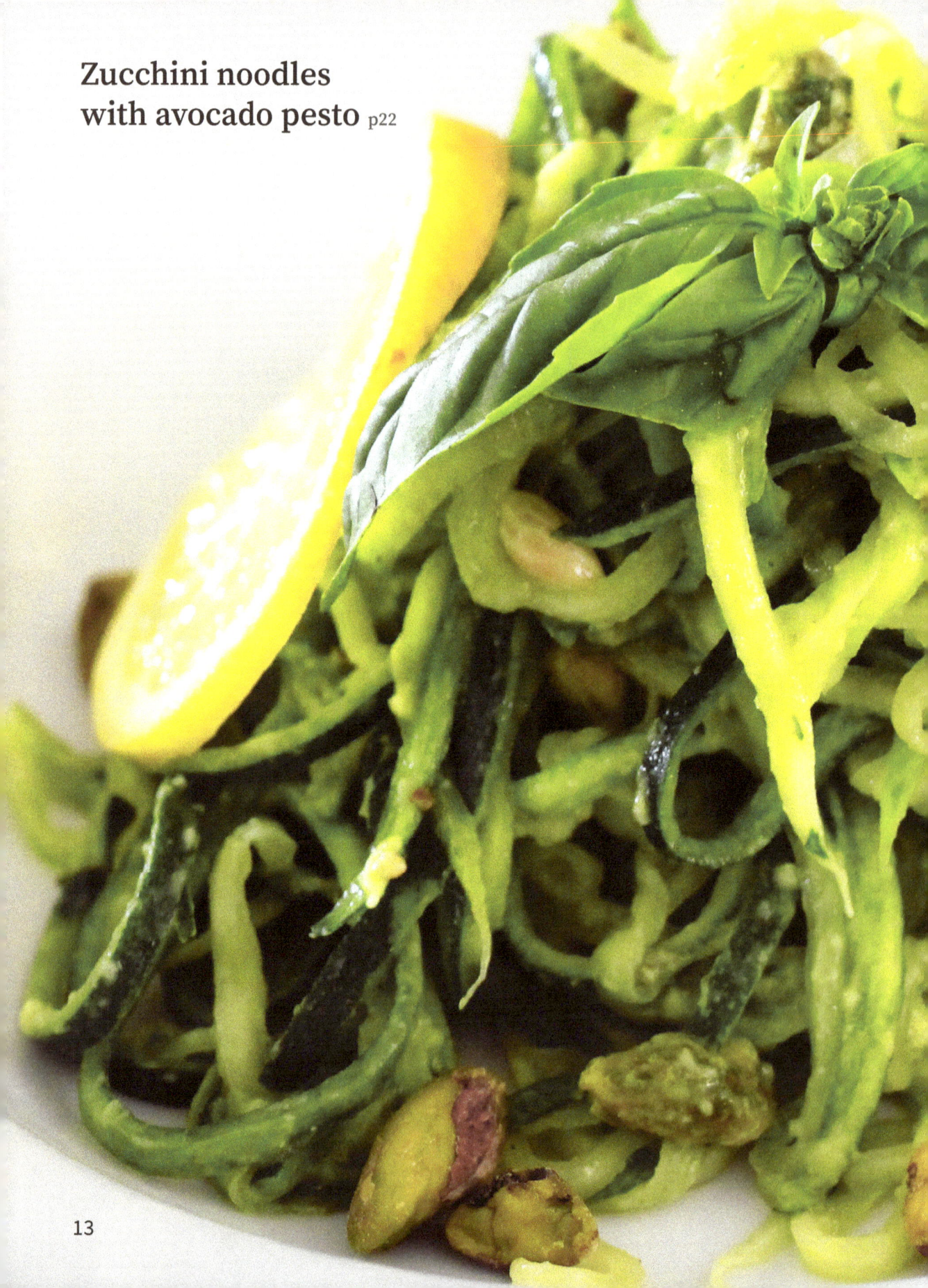

Zucchini noodles with avocado pesto p22

A Little Something on the side

Keep a few of these in the fridge and you'll never go hungry!

Low thiol vegetable stock	16	Fermented veg	24
Minted potato salad	17	Ginger infused rice	25
Asian vegetable salad	18	Carrots with honey orange glaze	26
Low thiol Thai curry paste	20	Asian style dumplings	27
Skordalia	21	Spiced roast pumpkin	29
Zucchini noodles with avocado pesto	22	Lemon & basil infused rice	30

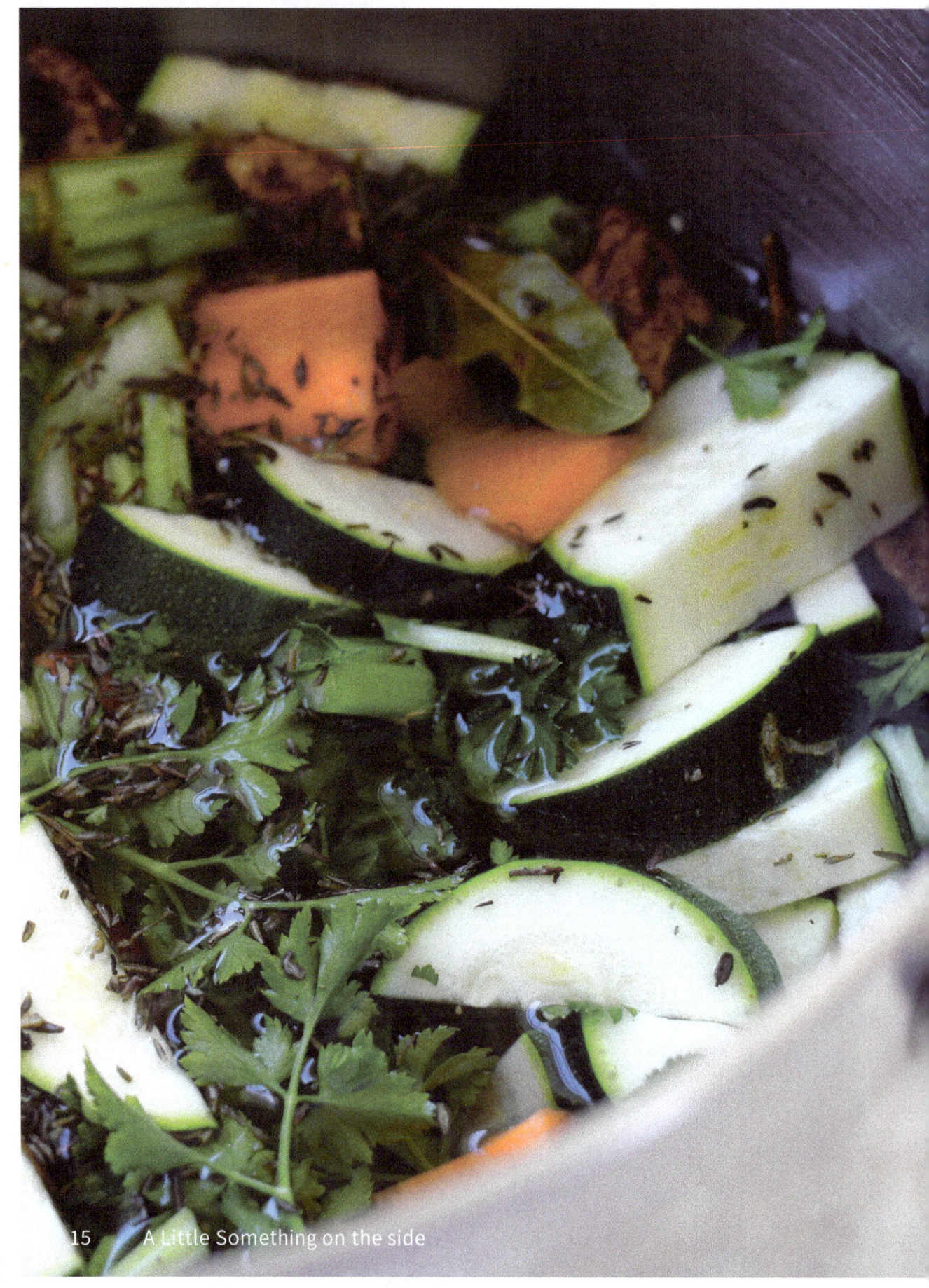

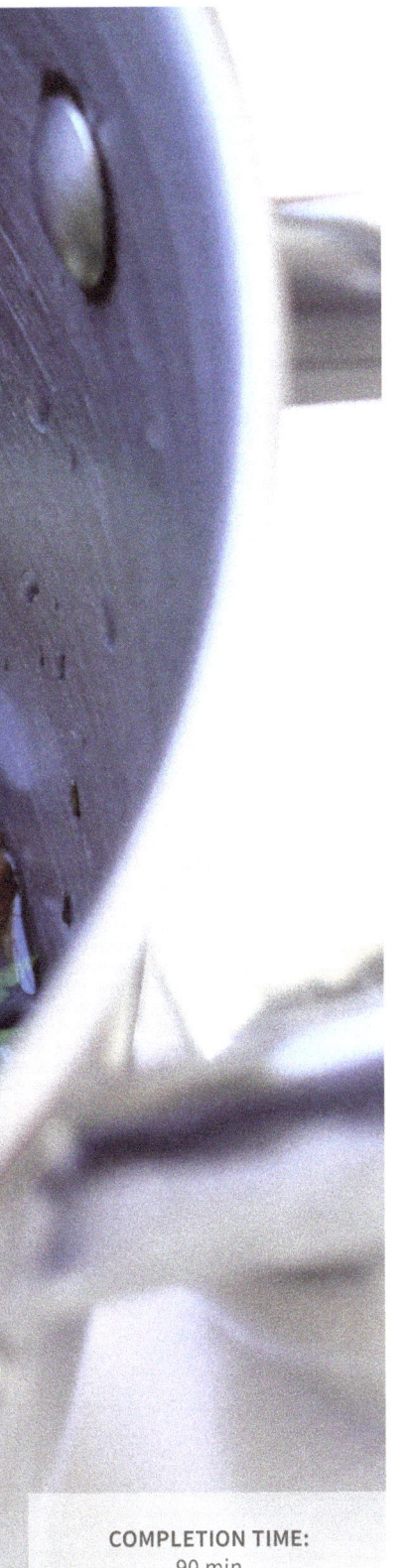

Low thiol vegetable stock

Gluten Free · Nut Free · Vegetarian · Dairy Free · Sugar Free

Ingredients

- celery
- parsnip
- fennel bulb
- sweet potato
- carrots
- zucchini
- 2 tsp asafoetida
- bay leaves
- parsley
- rosemary
- thyme
- himalayan salt
- ground pepper
- 2 L pure filtered water free of chlorine and fluoride

Method

1. Place the peeled and chopped vegetables into a large saucepan of pure filtered water together with the rosemary and thyme. Bring to the boil then cover and simmer slowly for 40 minutes.
2. Add the chopped parsley for the final 2 minutes
3. Add salt and pepper to your taste
4. Allow to cool then strain and keep in an airtight container for up to 4 days in the fridge or freeze for longer

COMPLETION TIME: 90 min

LEVEL: Easy

PREP: 10 min

YIELD: 4 - 6 servings

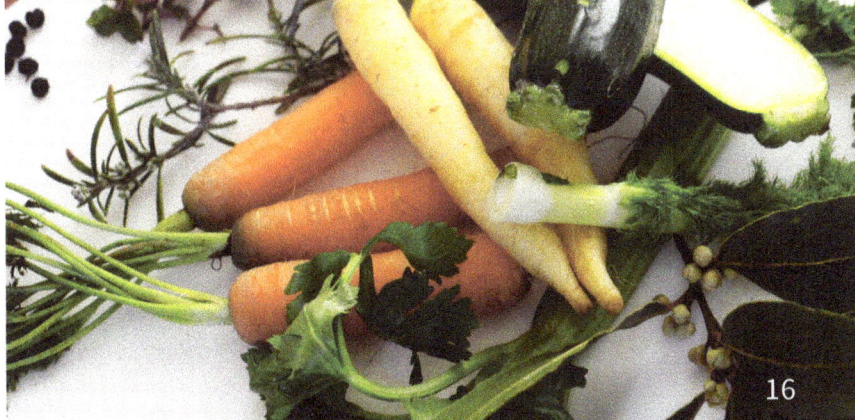

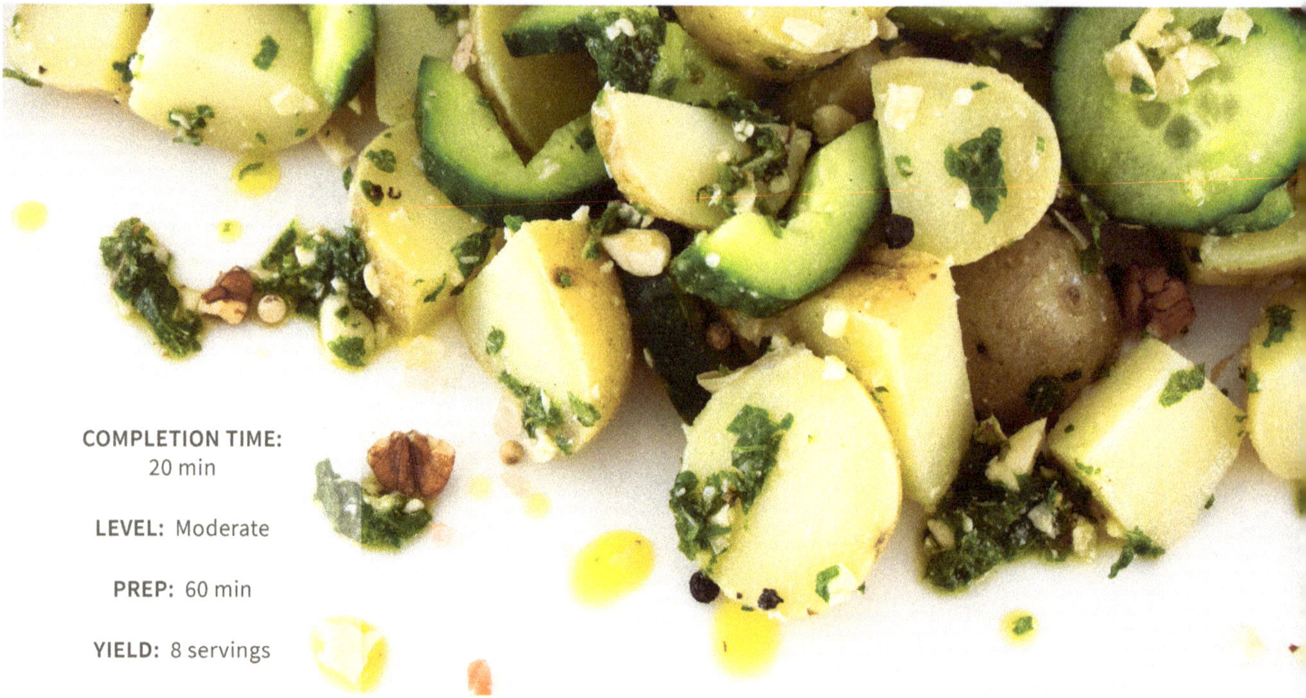

COMPLETION TIME: 20 min

LEVEL: Moderate

PREP: 60 min

YIELD: 8 servings

Minted potato salad

Gluten Free   Vegetarian   Dairy Free   Sugar Free

Choose from as wide a variety of vegetables as possible including varieties of potatoes. The greater the plant-food diversity the greater the microbial diversity in your digestive system. The more colour you can add to your diet the higher the polyphenol content of the diet. This too will promote the growth of protective microbes. Look for purple, red and orange varieties including sweet potato varieties. Serving cooked potato chilled increases the levels of resistant starch which is another great way to boost friendly gut bugs.

Ingredients

1kg new potatoes

250g of cucumber seeds removed and diced

1 cup mint leaves

1/4 cup blanched almonds, toasted

2 Tbs of walnut or hazelnut oil

1 Tbs of white wine vinegar

salt and pepper

Method

1. Place the potatoes in a saucepan of cold water and add a little salt. Bring to the boil and cook for 20 minutes or until tender
2. Drain and allow to cool
3. While the potatoes are cooking place the mint, toasted almonds, oil, and vinegar into a food processor and process to desired consistency
4. Combine potatoes, cucumber, salt, pepper, and mint pesto in a large bowl
5. Dress and Serve

Asian vegetable salad

Gluten Free   Nut Free   Dairy Free

This recipe can be varied to your tastes by adding or subtracting animal protein. Mineral transport can be significantly disturbed by heavy metals. Boosting mineral content with foods such as sea vegetables and anchovies also boosts flavour.

Ingredients

- 1 small head butter lettuce
- 1/2 cup bamboo shoots
- 1/2 cup julienne carrots
- 1/2 cup julienne cucumber
- 1/2 cup julienne red pepper
- 1/2 cup halved cherry tomatoes
- 1 finely shredded kaffir lime leaf
- 1/4 cup shredded mint leaves
- 1/4 cup Thai basil leaves
- 1 Tbs fresh lime juice
- 2 tsp fish sauce
- 1 tsp coco aminos
- 1 Tbs sesame oil
- 1 tsp rapadura or coconut sugar
- 2 tsp dried anchovies fried in coconut oil

Method

1. Place all vegetable ingredients including the basil, mint and kaffir lime leaves into a salad bowl
2. Mix the lime juice, fish sauce, sesame oil, coco aminos and sugar together and toss through the salad
3. Serve topped with a sprinkling of fried anchovies

Variation: 1/2 cup of shredded cooked chicken or duck or strips of seared beef may be added.

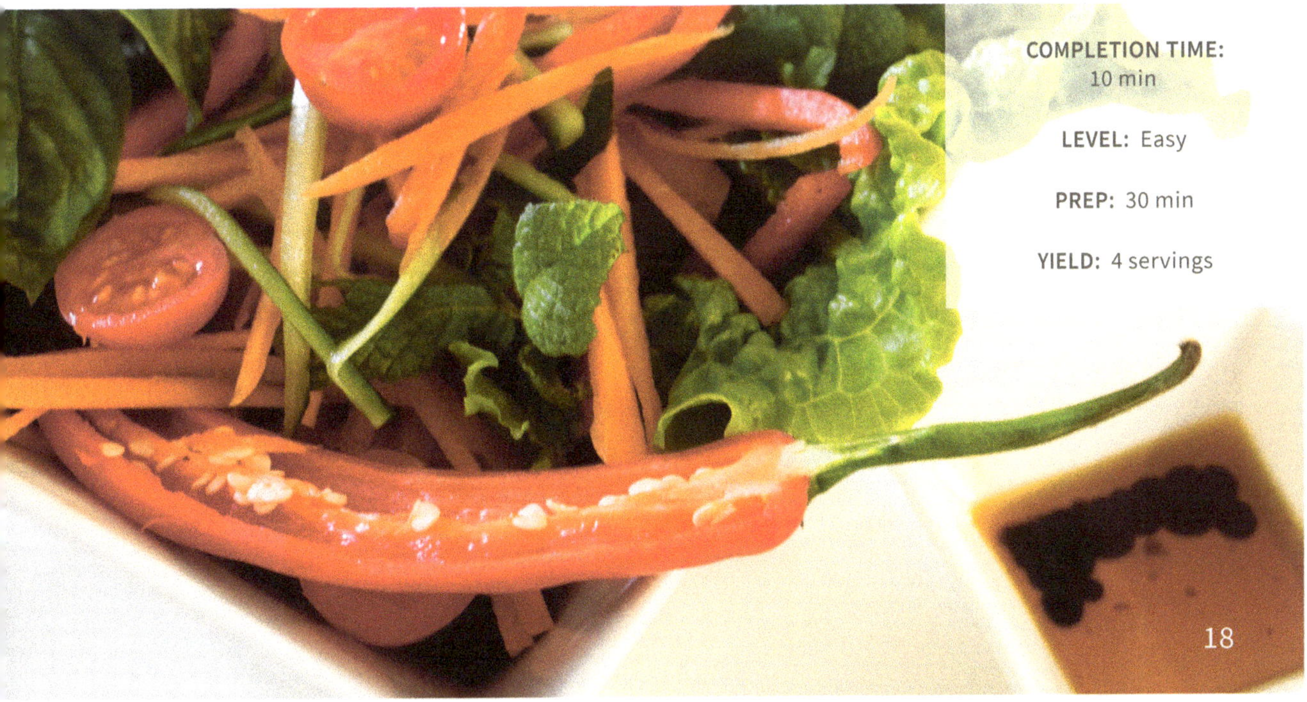

COMPLETION TIME: 10 min

LEVEL: Easy

PREP: 30 min

YIELD: 4 servings

COMPLETION TIME:
15 min

LEVEL: Easy

PREP: 15 min

YIELD: 4 servings

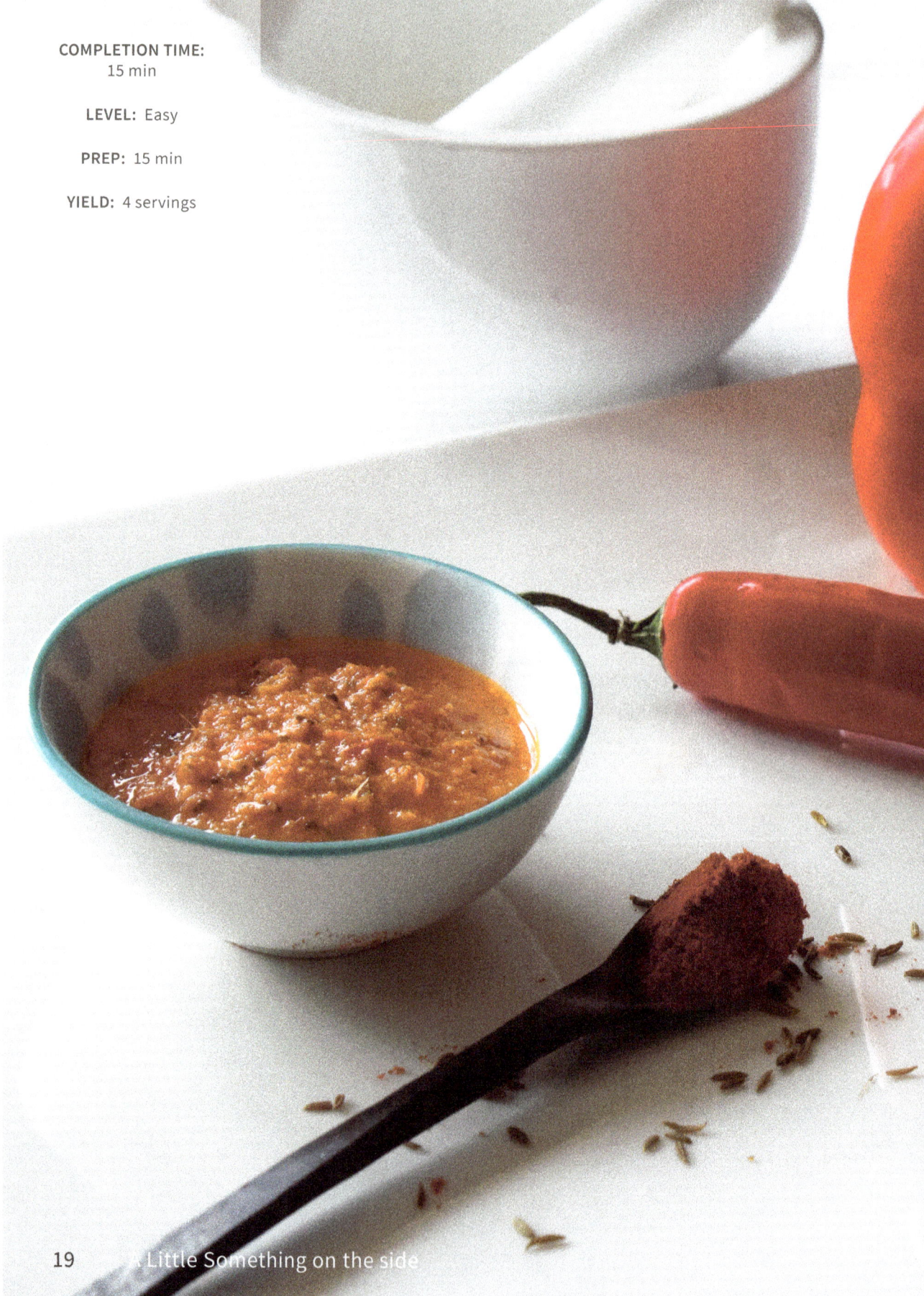

Low thiol Thai curry paste

Gluten Free · Nut Free · Vegetarian · Sugar Free

Ingredients

2 Tbs organic cold-pressed olive oil

3 cm piece fresh ginger sliced

1 tsp asafoetida

2 large mild red chillies with the seeds removed

2 lemon grass stalks - use the inner tender portion

2 tsp Thai basil

1 tsp ground cumin

1 tsp paprika

1/2 large red capsicum (pepper) seeds removed and sliced

1 tsp Himalayan salt

ground pepper to taste

Method

1. Place the above ingredients into food processor and blend to a smooth consistency. Add a little more oil as needed to allow the machine to run. You may need to use a tamper (suitable for your machine) to push the ingredients down to the blade

Note: This paste will keep for around 5 days in a sealed glass jar in the fridge.

Resuscitating Thai curry
Page 64

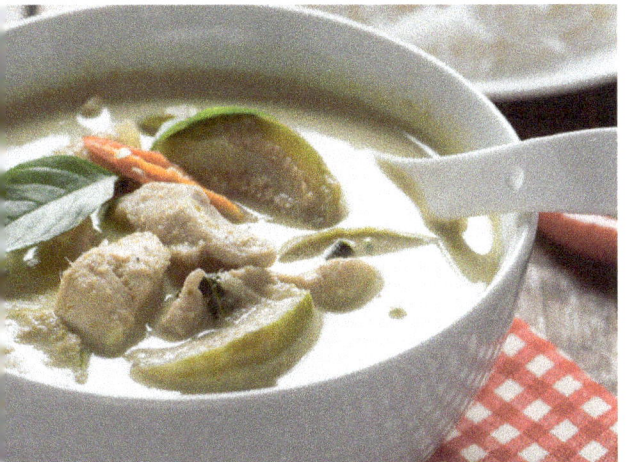

Thai-style fish curry
Page 41

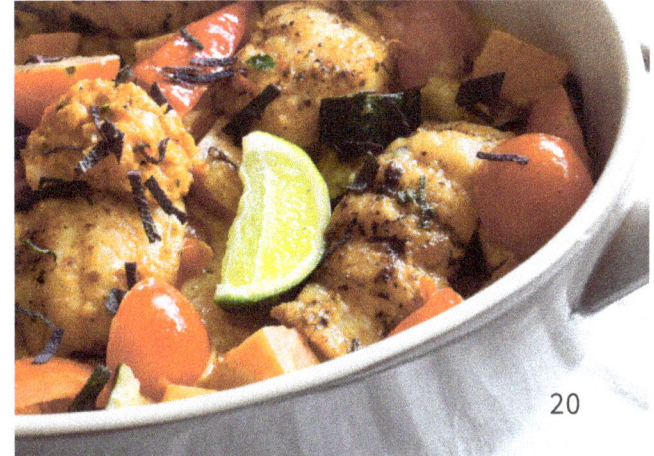

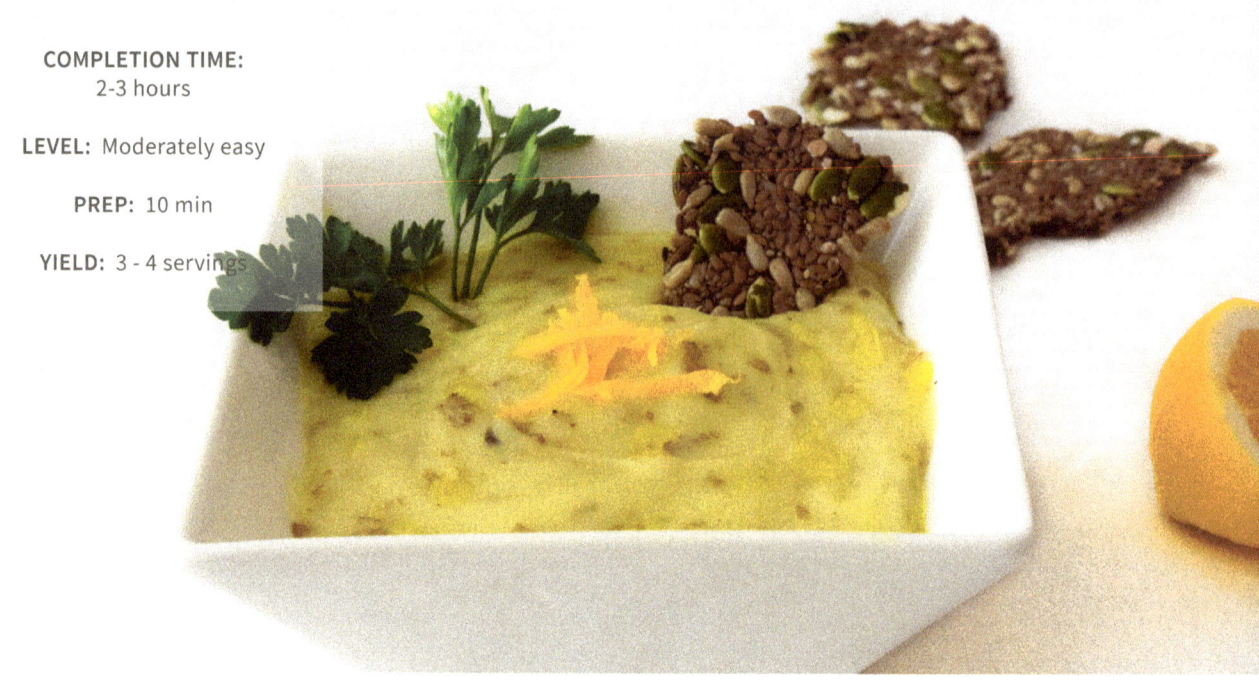

COMPLETION TIME: 2-3 hours

LEVEL: Moderately easy

PREP: 10 min

YIELD: 3 - 4 servings

Skordalia

 Gluten Free   Nut Free   Vegetarian   Sugar Free

Chilling cooked root vegetables converts the starches to resistant or retrograde starch which provides fuel for your microbiota- the beneficial bugs which live in your digestive tract and help to protect against heavy metal absorption.

Ingredients

5 small floury* potatoes unpeeled
1 Tbs extra virgin olive oil
1 tsp chopped parsley
pinch of salt
squeeze of fresh lemon juice
1/4 tsp asafoetida
extra oil to serve

*Floury potatoes: King Edward, Desiree, Dutch Cream, Kipfler, Nicola.

Method

1. Cook and drain the potatoes. Mash
2. Place potatoes into a food processor along with the chopped parsley, salt, olive oil, lemon juice and the asafoetida. Process until smooth
3. Transfer into a dish and press down
4. Refrigerate until thoroughly chilled
5. Serve as a dip or a side topped with lemon zest and a drizzle of oil

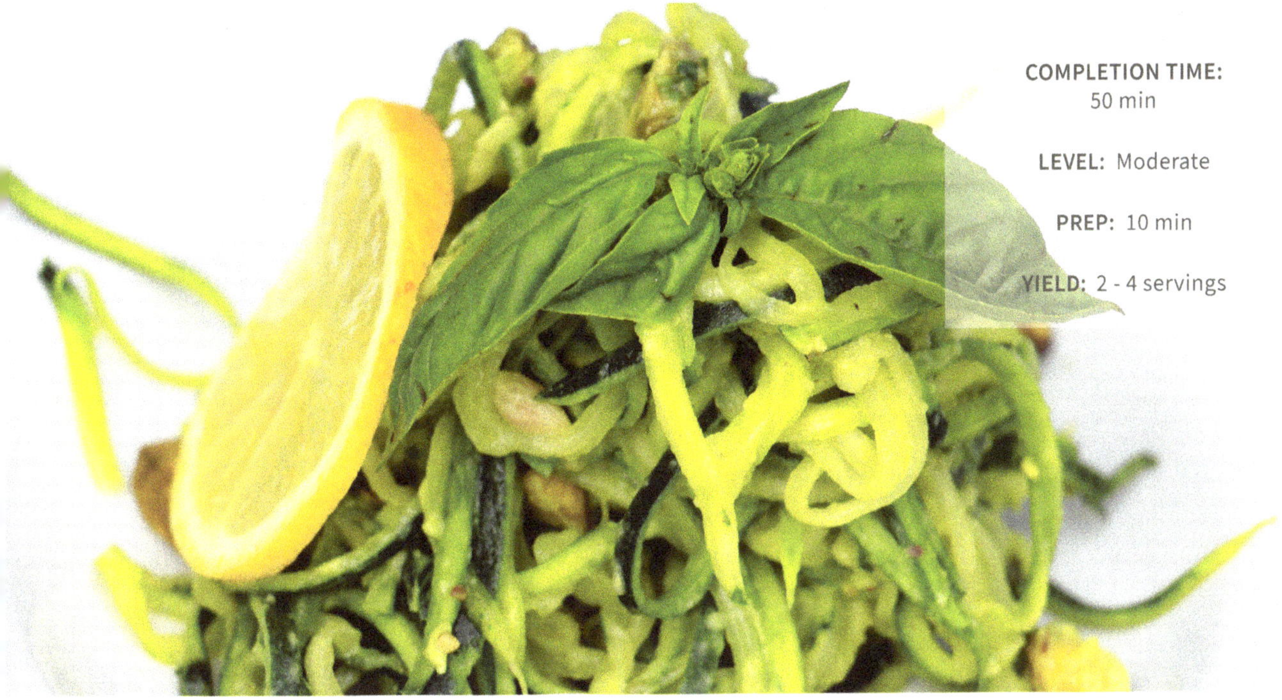

COMPLETION TIME: 50 min

LEVEL: Moderate

PREP: 10 min

YIELD: 2 - 4 servings

Zucchini noodles with avocado pesto

 Gluten Free   Vegetarian   Dairy Free   Sugar Free

Ingredients

6 medium zucchini, ends trimmed
1/2 tsp salt
1 large ripe avocado
1 cup basil leaves
1/2 cup activated*and dried unsalted shelled pistachios
2 Tbs lemon juice
pinch ground pepper
2 Tbs avocado oil
1/4 tsp salt extra

Method

1. Prepare the zucchini using a vegetable peeler, mandolin, or spiral vegetable slicer. Discard the seeds when you reach the middle as they make the noodles fall apart
2. Put the zucchini noodles into a colander and mix with the salt and allow to drain for about 30 minutes. Squeeze noodles gently to remove any excess moisture
3. Place the avocado, basil, pistachios, lemon juice, pepper and avocado oil and remaining salt into a food processor and blend until smooth
4. Add a little avocado oil to a pan and add the zucchini noodles, warm for about 5 minutes and gently mix through the avocado pesto
5. Serve warm topped with a sprig of fresh basil and a drizzle of oil

*For more information about why it is important to activate and dry nuts, see page xxiv

A Little Something on the side

COMPLETION TIME:
1-3 weeks

LEVEL: Moderate

PREP: 60 min

YIELD: 4 servings

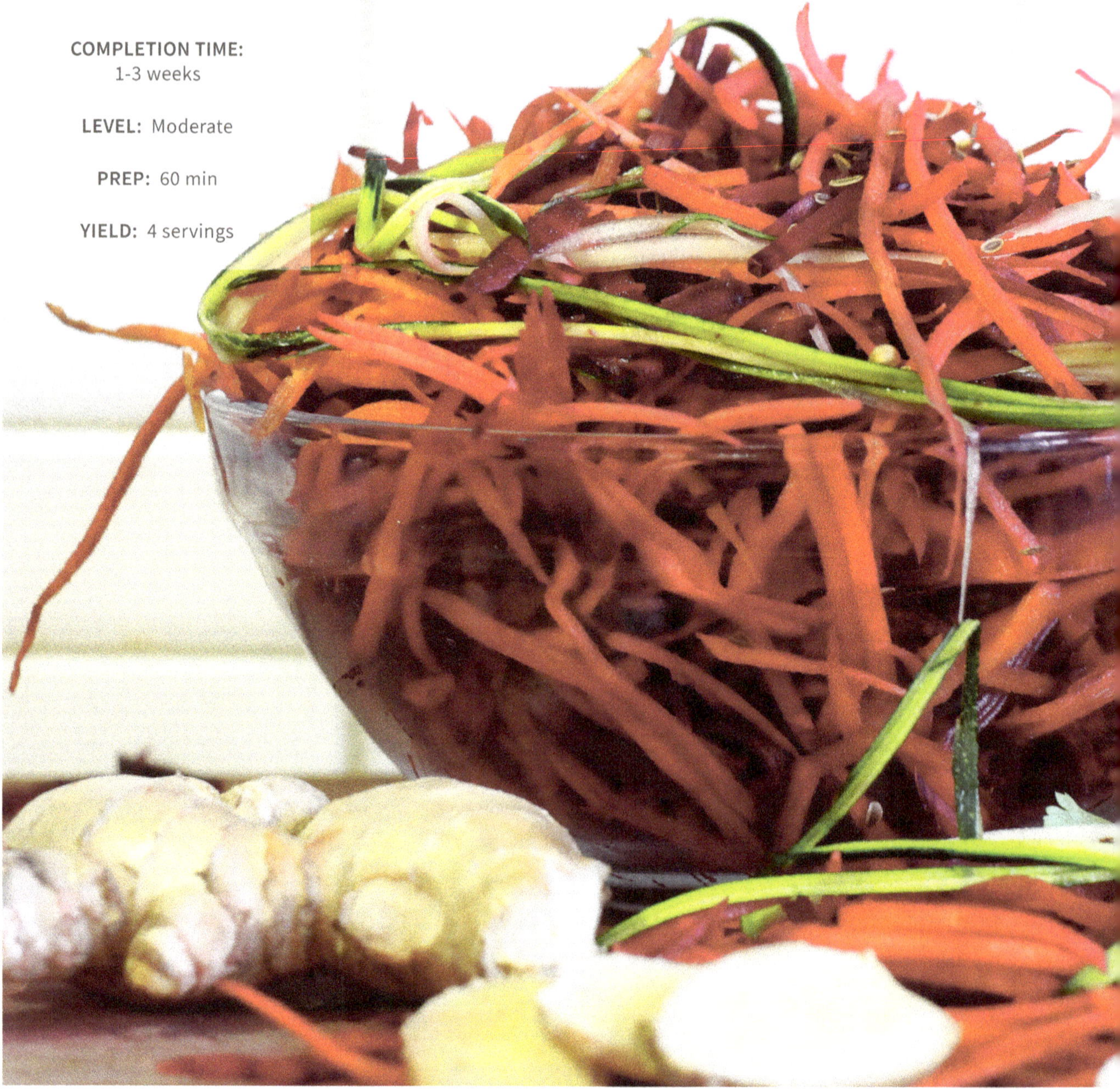

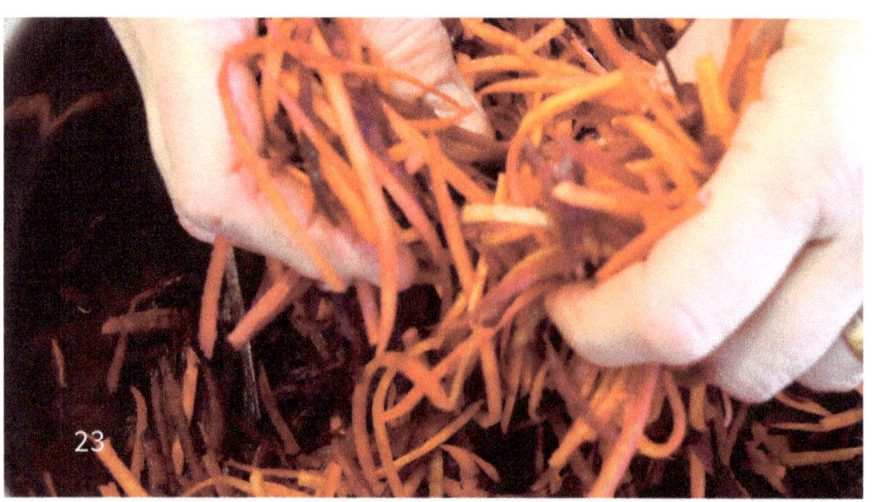
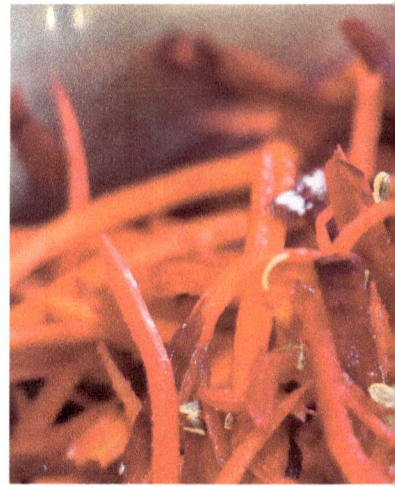

Fermented veg

Gluten Free   Nut Free   Vegetarian   Sugar Free

Live cultured foods support a healthy gut microbial population thus limiting the reabsorption of metals via the gut wall. Including fermented foods daily especially with cooked meats will provide digestive enzymes which are often depleted by heavy metals.

Ingredients

Equal quantities of the following vegetables;
beetroot
zucchini
carrot

A 5 - 10 cm piece of ginger roughly chopped

1 Tbs of salt per 2kg of vegetables

1 Tbs of caraway or dill seeds per 2kg of vegetables

2 Tbs of prepared *Kombucha* (p93) per kg of vegetables. Shop bought is fine - choose original or ginger flavour

Method

1. Top and tail the vegetables as needed, there's no need to peel them
2. Grate or shred the vegetables into a large bowl together with the kombucha
3. In a mortar and Pestle grind the ginger, spices and salt and add to the vegetables
4. Crush the vegetables with your hands until they feel juicy or use a wooden kraut pounder
5. Place into a fermenting crock or pickl'it airlock jars
6. Place the stones on top to weigh the vegetables below the liquid and fill the crock moat or air lock with water to keep air out and facilitate an anaerobic process
7. Listen to your ferment as it slowly increases gas production- it will bubble and gurgle. When this begins to slow your ferment is ready to be transferred into jars and stored in the refrigerator

A Little Something on the side

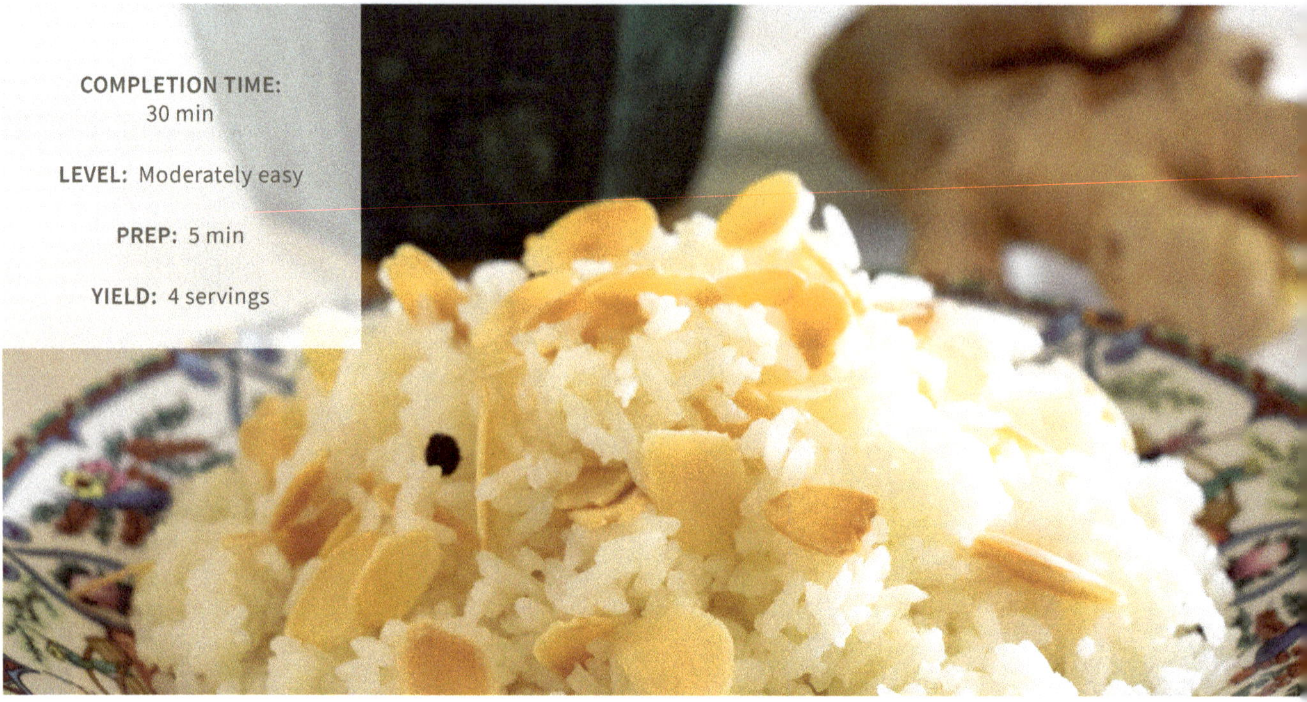

COMPLETION TIME:
30 min

LEVEL: Moderately easy

PREP: 5 min

YIELD: 4 servings

Ginger infused rice

Gluten Free   Vegetarian   Dairy Free   Sugar Free

Ingredients

1 cup basmati rice
1 1/2 cups water
1/2 tsp shredded or grated ginger
2 Tbs toasted slithered almonds

Method

1. Add rice, water and ginger to a saucepan and seal with a well fitted lid. Ensure that the water level is 1 1/2 cm above the rice
2. Bring to the boil then reduce to a medium heat and cook for approx. 10 minutes until the liquid has been absorbed and the rice is tender
3. Stir through the almonds
4. Serve with your choice of protein or vegetable

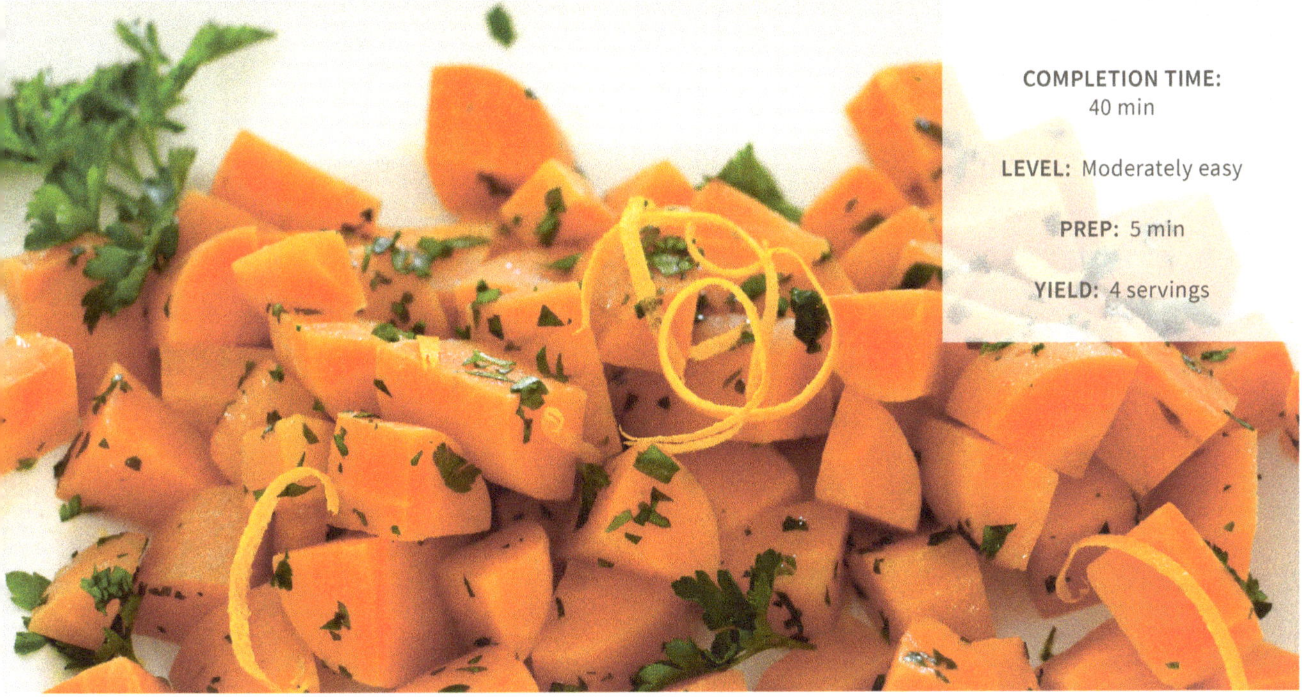

COMPLETION TIME: 40 min

LEVEL: Moderately easy

PREP: 5 min

YIELD: 4 servings

Carrots with honey orange glaze

Gluten Free | Nut Free | Vegetarian | Dairy Free | Sugar Free

Ingredients

1/4 cup parsley (fresh, finely chopped)

1 Tbs orange juice (freshly squeezed and a little zest)

8 carrots (medium, organic)

2 Tbs organic ghee

1/2 tsp of honey

Method

1. Wash carrots and trim the ends. Cut each carrot lengthwise and then cut diagonally at about 2 cm intervals
2. Place carrots in pan and cover with filtered water. Cover pan and cook to desired tenderness
3. Drain carrots and set aside
4. Place ghee in the warm pan and melt on low heat. Add the orange juice, grated orange zest and honey to taste
5. Place the carrots back in the pan and toss in the orange butter. Turn off the heat, add the parsley, toss again and serve immediately

Asian style dumplings

Gluten Free   Nut Free   Dairy Free   Sugar Free

Ingredients

Wrapper
1 cup white rice flour
1/2 cup tapioca flour
extra tapioca to flour the work surface and your hands
1 cup boiling water
1/2 tsp salt

Sauce
2 Tbs reduced* *Stock (p40)*
1/4 tsp ginger (finely chopped)
1 tsp rice vinegar
1 tsp cornstarch
1 tsp Himalayan salt
2 tsp chopped anchovies in olive oil

Filling
1 cup chopped mushrooms
1 cup shredded carrots
2 cups finely chopped celery

Method

Wrapper
1. Combine all of the ingredients in a bowl. Mix/knead to form a slightly sticky dough then turn out onto a tapioca-floured surface. Cover with a damp cloth and allow to rest for 15 minutes. Sprinkle with more tapioca and need once more and form into a ball. Dust your hands with tapioca and roll out a quarter of the dough into a 3 cm thick sausage shape. Use a sharp knife to divide each sausage into 4 equal pieces and form into balls
2. Roll out each piece as thinly as possible between two sheets of wax paper which have been lightly rubbed with tapioca. Stack the rolled wrappers in a bowl with wax paper between each. Cover the bowl with a wet towel. This will keep them from drying out whilst you prepare the rest

Sauce
3. Combine all the ingredients in a jar and shake

Filling
4. Add the veggies to a non-stick skillet over medium high heat. Once they begin to sizzle, add about 1/3 cup of water or stock, cover the pan, and let them steam for 4-5 minutes over medium heat until soft
5. Remove the cover, add the sauce mixture, and stir until everything comes together and all additional liquid has evaporated. About 1-2 minutes. Remove from heat and allow to cool for 5-10 minutes

To assemble
1. Remove one wrapper from the bowl together with the waxed paper
2. Spoon about a teaspoon of filling into the centre of the wrapper. Fold in half and press the edges together firmly
3. Draw the free edge together to form a dumpling shape pinching the free edge closed as you go
4. Keep your hands dry and lightly dusted throughout
5. Repeat with the remaining wrappers

To steam
6. Fill a shallow pan with enough water to completely cover the bottom. Bring to a boil. Add half of your dumplings. Cover and steam for 5-6 minutes. Remove from the pan. Repeat with the second half
7. Serve with broth or try them deep fried in a blend of ghee and coconut oil until crisp and lightly browned

*NOTE: Stock can be reduced by boiling the uncovered, strained liquid rapidly until it reduces down to the desired quantity or consistency. This is how great sauces are made. Avoid leaving the pot unattended.

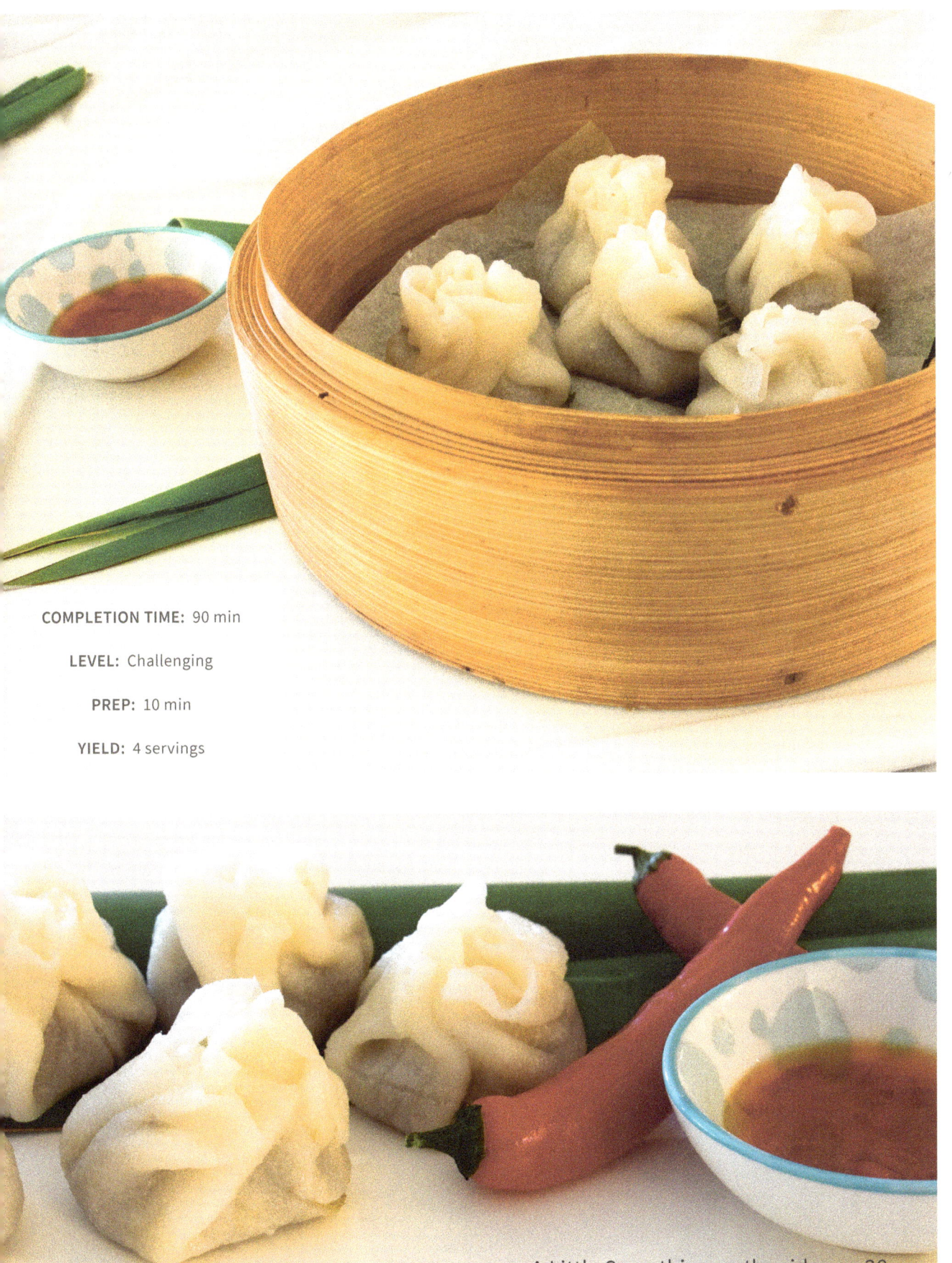

COMPLETION TIME: 90 min

LEVEL: Challenging

PREP: 10 min

YIELD: 4 servings

A Little Something on the side

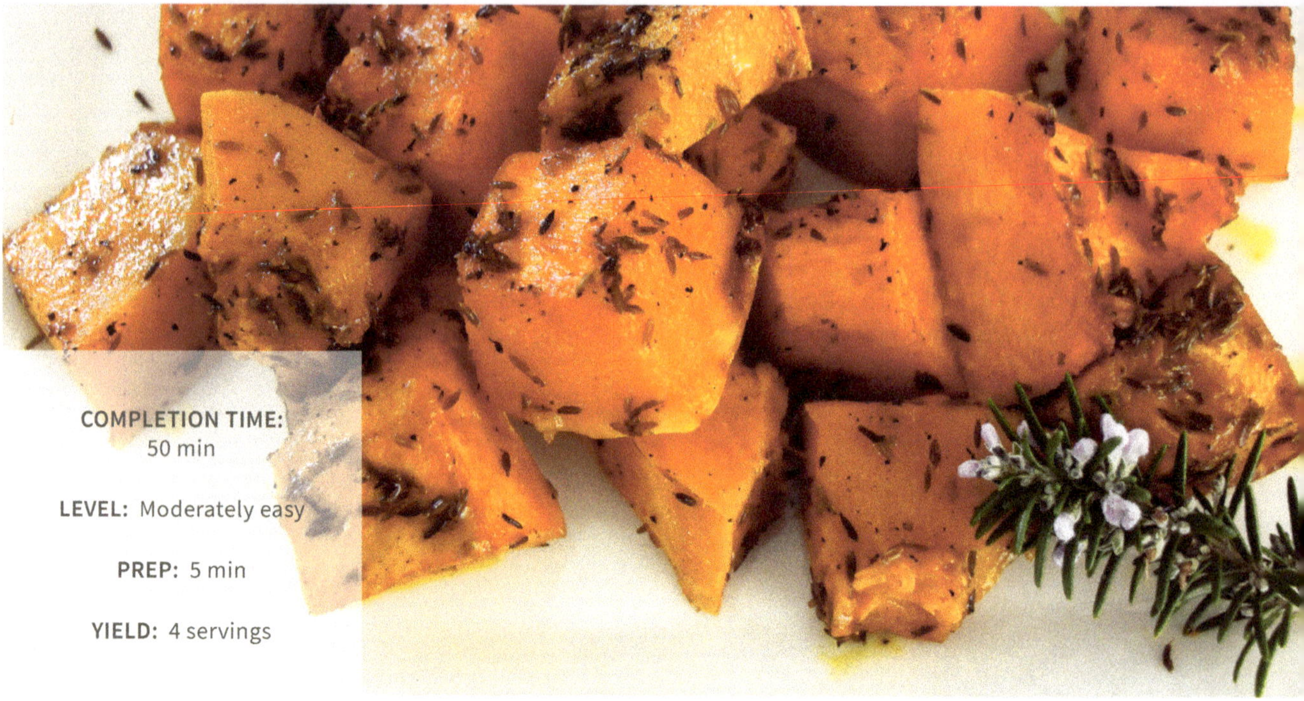

COMPLETION TIME: 50 min

LEVEL: Moderately easy

PREP: 5 min

YIELD: 4 servings

Spiced roast pumpkin

Gluten Free | Nut Free | Vegetarian | Dairy Free | Sugar Free

Adding good quality fats or oil to dishes which contain vegetables is not only for flavour but also for nutritional emphasis as fats increase the bioavailability of phytonutrients.

Ingredients

1 tsp sea salt

2 cups Japanese pumpkin (diced)

1 Tbs ghee

1 tsp cumin seeds

pinch of freshly grated nutmeg

Method

1. Pre-heat oven to 180°C or 350°F
2. Cut the pumpkin into evenly sized chunks
3. Sprinkle with the cumin seeds nutmeg and salt and drizzle with melted ghee or butter
4. Stir to combine, ensuring that all the pumpkin chunks are evenly covered
5. Roast for 30 minutes, or until the pumpkin is golden brown and cooked through

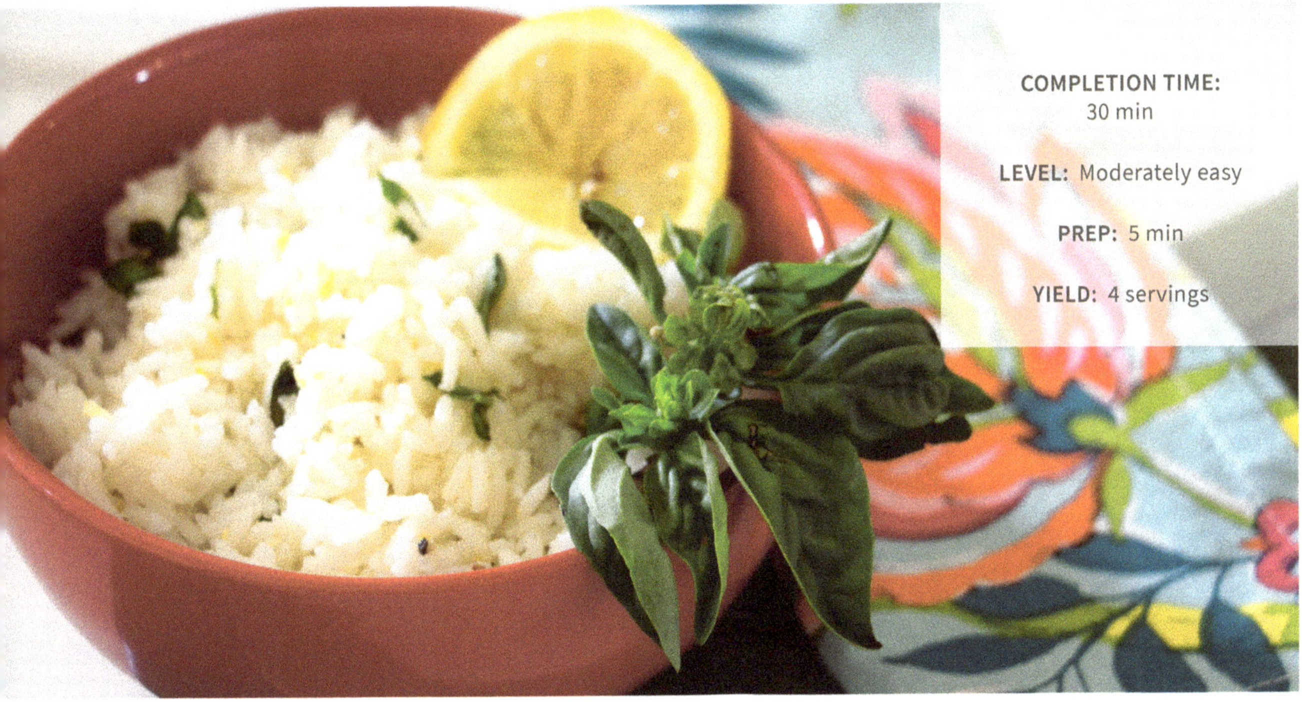

COMPLETION TIME: 30 min

LEVEL: Moderately easy

PREP: 5 min

YIELD: 4 servings

Lemon & basil infused rice

Gluten Free | Nut Free | Vegetarian | Dairy Free | Sugar Free

Ingredients

1 cup basmati rice

1 1/2 cups *Low thiol vegetable stock* *(p16)*
Ensure that the stock level is 1 1/2 cm above the rice

1 Tbs grated lemon zest

salt and pepper to season

1/3 cup shredded basil

Method

1. Place rice, vegetable stock and grated lemon zest into a saucepan and bring to the boil. Reduce to a gentle or medium heat until almost all of the liquid has been absorbed
2. Remove the saucepan from the heat and season with salt and pepper and mix through the shredded basil
3. Serve with wild caught fish* or vegetables

**NOTE: Farmed fish may be a source of antibiotic and in the case of some farmed Salmon artificial colours. Choose smaller, wild caught fish avoiding any fish with a fillet size large than a dinner plate. Avoid fish known to contain higher levels of mercury such as Ling, Tuna, Shark, Swordfish, King Mackerel, Marlin, Tilefish.*

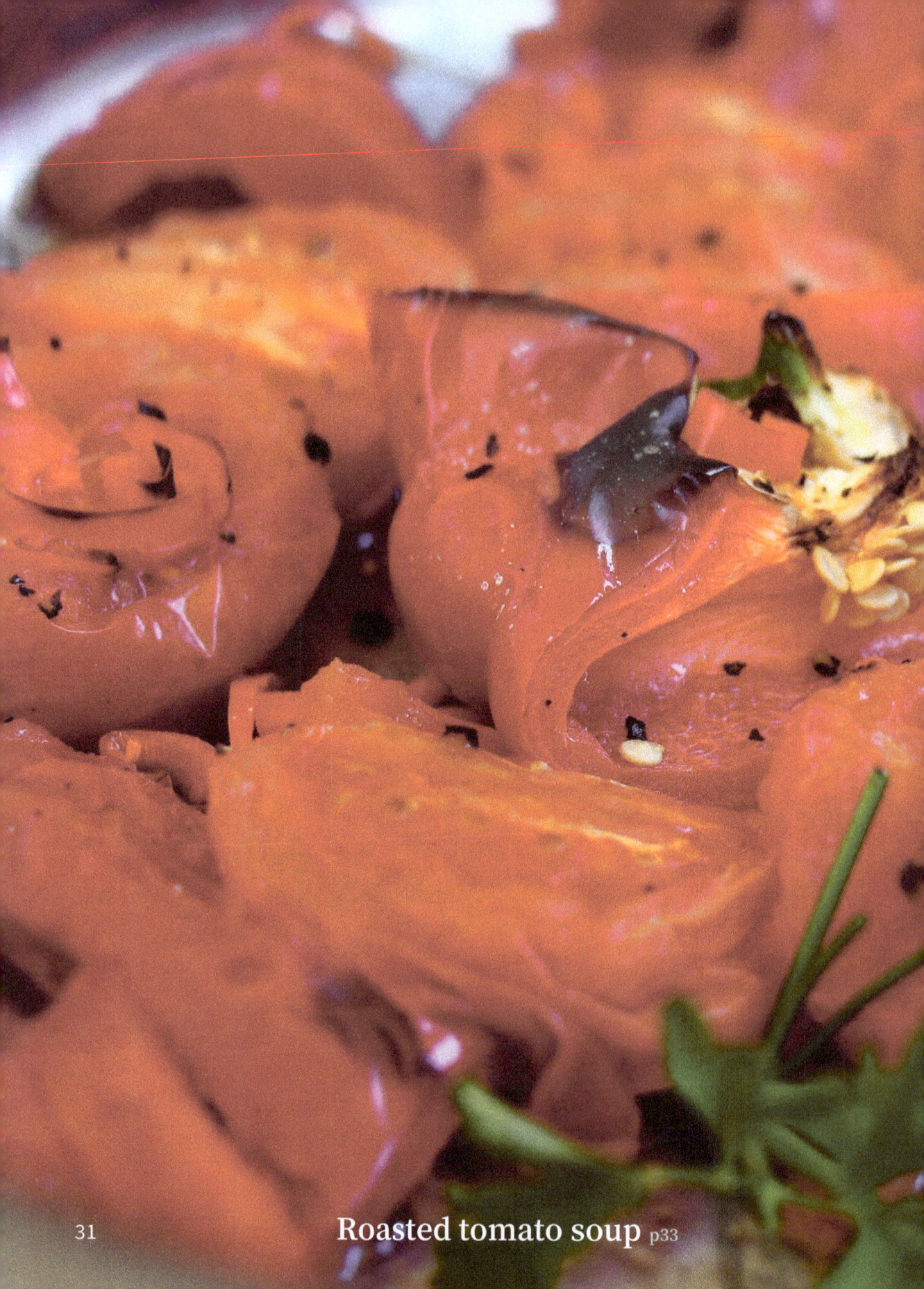

Roasted tomato soup p33

Warm Your ♥ Heart Soups

To thaw your fingers & toes

Roasted tomato soup	33	Mediterranean seafood soup	35
Vegetable soup	34	Poultry soup	36

COMPLETION TIME: 60 min

LEVEL: Easy

PREP: 15 min

YIELD: 4 servings

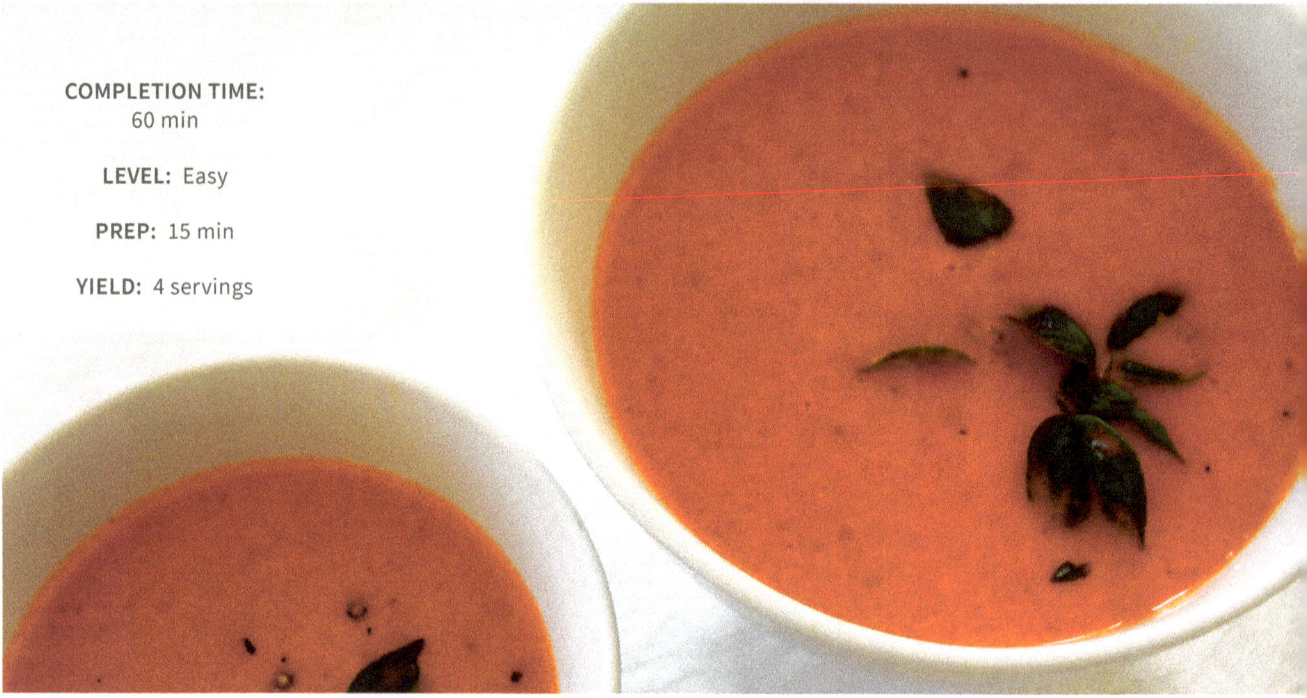

Roasted tomato soup

Gluten Free — Nut Free — Vegetarian — Dairy Free — Sugar Free

Ingredients

10 ripe Roma tomatoes halved

2 large red capsicum sliced

3 chillies finely chopped

1 Tbs fresh oregano

1 Tbs olive oil

4 cups of chicken *(p40)* or vegetable stock *(p16)* (vegetarian option use only vegetable stock)

1 cup coconut (nut-free option) or almond milk

salt and pepper to season

1 Tbs shredded basil leaves

Method

1. Place capsicum, chillies and tomatoes cut side up on baking tray. Drizzle with the oil and season with salt and pepper. Roast for about 30 minutes at 180°C or 350°F until the tomato softens

2. In a large saucepan add the roasted tomato, capsicum and chilli together with the stock and slowly bring to the boil, reduce heat and simmer gently for about 10 minutes or until the soup thickens slightly. Add the coconut or almond milk and blend with a stick blender to the desired consistency. Take care blending hot foods

3. Season with salt and pepper, sprinkle with shredded basil leaves

4. Serve

Note: For vegetarian/vegan option use vegetable stock

Vegetable soup

Gluten Free   Nut Free   Vegetarian   Dairy Free   Sugar Free

Ingredients

- 4 celery stalks chopped
- 1 red capsicum (pepper) diced
- 1 green capsicum (pepper) diced
- 4 carrots chopped
- 2 parsnips chopped
- 2 large potatoes diced
- 1/2 butternut pumpkin diced
- 2 large zucchini diced
- 1/2 tsp salt
- Pinch ground pepper
- Dash of Coco Amino sauce
- 1 Tbs thyme leaves
- 1 Tbs oregano leaves
- 1/2 cup chopped parsley
- 1 finely chopped chilli
- 1 grated apple if desired for a little sweetness
- 6 cups pure spring or filtered water*
- Himalayan salt and ground pepper to taste

*Option: Use chicken stock to replace water

Option: Add 1/2 cup of soaked and cooked red rice to thicken.

Method

1. Add all ingredients apart from fresh herbs to a large saucepan and bring to the boil. Reduce heat and simmer gently for 1 hour or until vegetables are the desired consistency
2. Alternatively all ingredients can be placed into a slow cooker on low setting and left to gently cook overnight

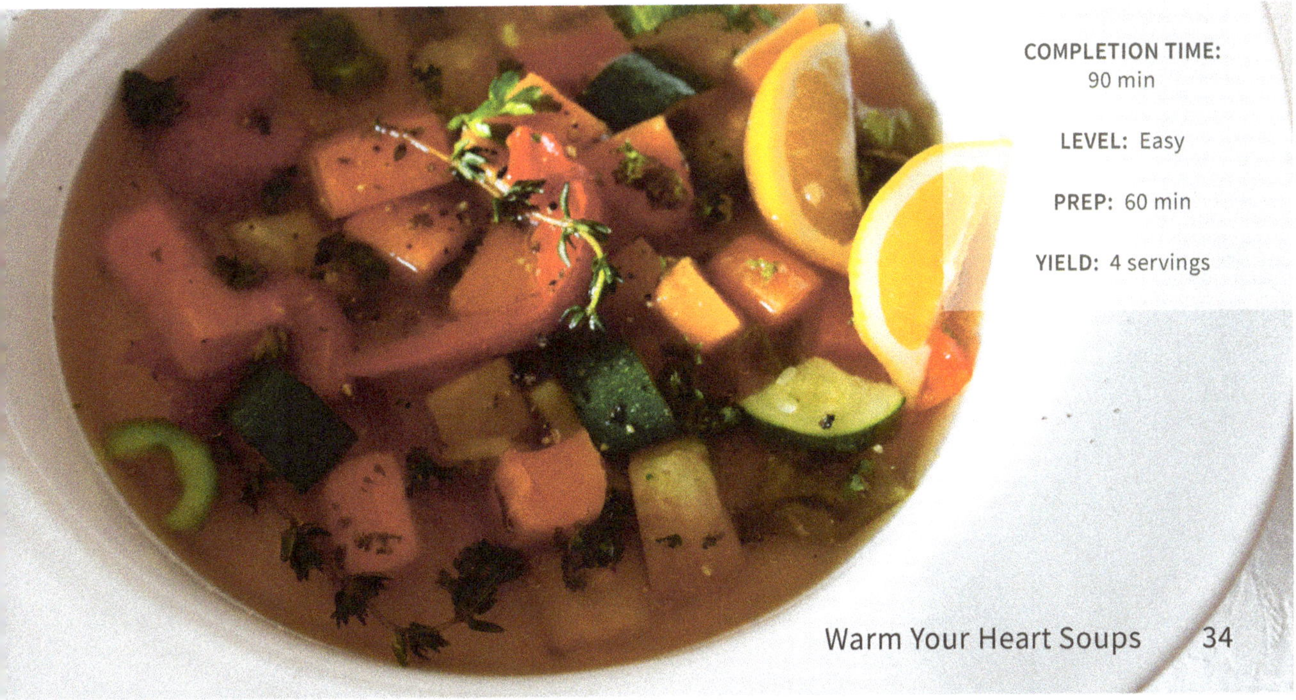

COMPLETION TIME: 90 min

LEVEL: Easy

PREP: 60 min

YIELD: 4 servings

Warm Your Heart Soups

Mediterranean seafood soup

Gluten Free Nut Free Dairy Free Sugar Free

Ingredients

1 green capsicum (pepper) deseeded and finely diced

1 red capsicum (pepper) deseeded and finely diced

4 medium tomatoes diced

1 1/2 cups fish, chicken *(p40)* or vegetable stock *(p16)*

5 strands saffron

1 Tbs fresh thyme

3 bay leaves

1/2 preserved lemon cut into strips

1kg skinless Hake cut into chunks

salt and pepper to taste

1/2 cup fresh basil leaves

3 anchovies and a little olive oil from the jar

1/2 cup green olives

Method

1. Add the capsicum, tomatoes, fish stock, saffron, thyme, bay leaves, anchovies, anchovy oil and preserved lemon into a large saucepan and slowly bring to the boil. Reduce heat and simmer for 15 to 20 minutes to allow the liquid to thicken

2. Add Hake chunks and cook for about 5 minutes or until the fish is just cooked. Add olives

3. Serve immediately, top with basil leaves, salt and pepper

Variation: For an added energy boost add 1 cup cooked red rice.

COMPLETION TIME: 30 min

LEVEL: Easy

PREP: 30 min

YIELD: 4 servings

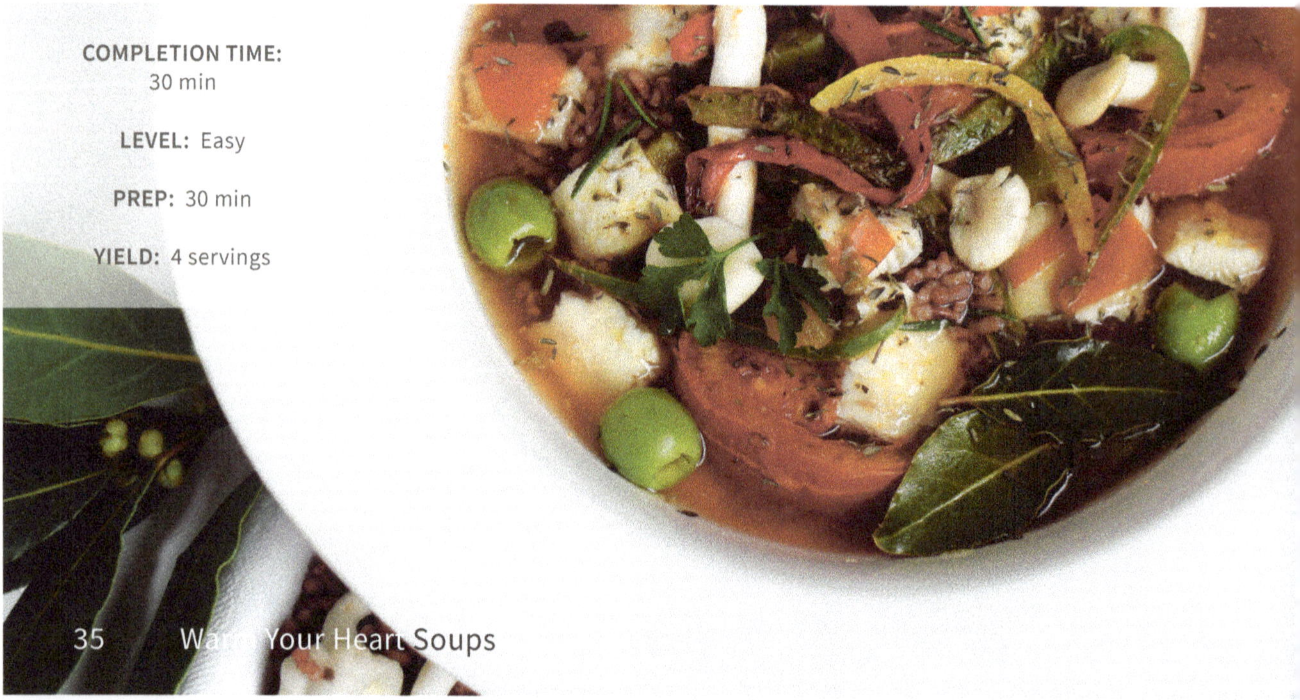

Poultry soup

Gluten Free Nut Free Dairy Free Sugar Free

Turkey is a rich source of tryptophan which the body can convert to serotonin and melatonin to aid mood and sleep. These neurotransmitters are often imbalanced in those with heavy metals toxicity.

Ingredients

1 whole organic chicken, duck or turkey, or chicken, duck or turkey pieces with bone in

3 celery stalks chopped

2 carrots diced

1/2 cup Shitaki mushrooms finely sliced

4 bay leaves

1 tsp thyme leaves

1/2 tsp salt

pepper to taste

5 cups of pure filtered water or sufficient to cover poultry

1/2 cup chopped parsley

1 Tbs lemon juice

Method

1. Add all ingredients except parsley and lemon juice to a slow cooker and cook on low setting overnight or for 10 - 12 hours
2. Remove poultry from cooker and discard bones. Shred flesh and return to soup
3. Add fresh parsley and a splash of lemon juice to serve
4. Store in the refrigerator for up to 4 days or freeze for longer

Option: For an Asian style soup omit the thyme leaves and add a 6 cm piece of chopped ginger, 1 Tbs five spice powder, the juice and zest of 1 orange, 1 Tbs of coco aminos.

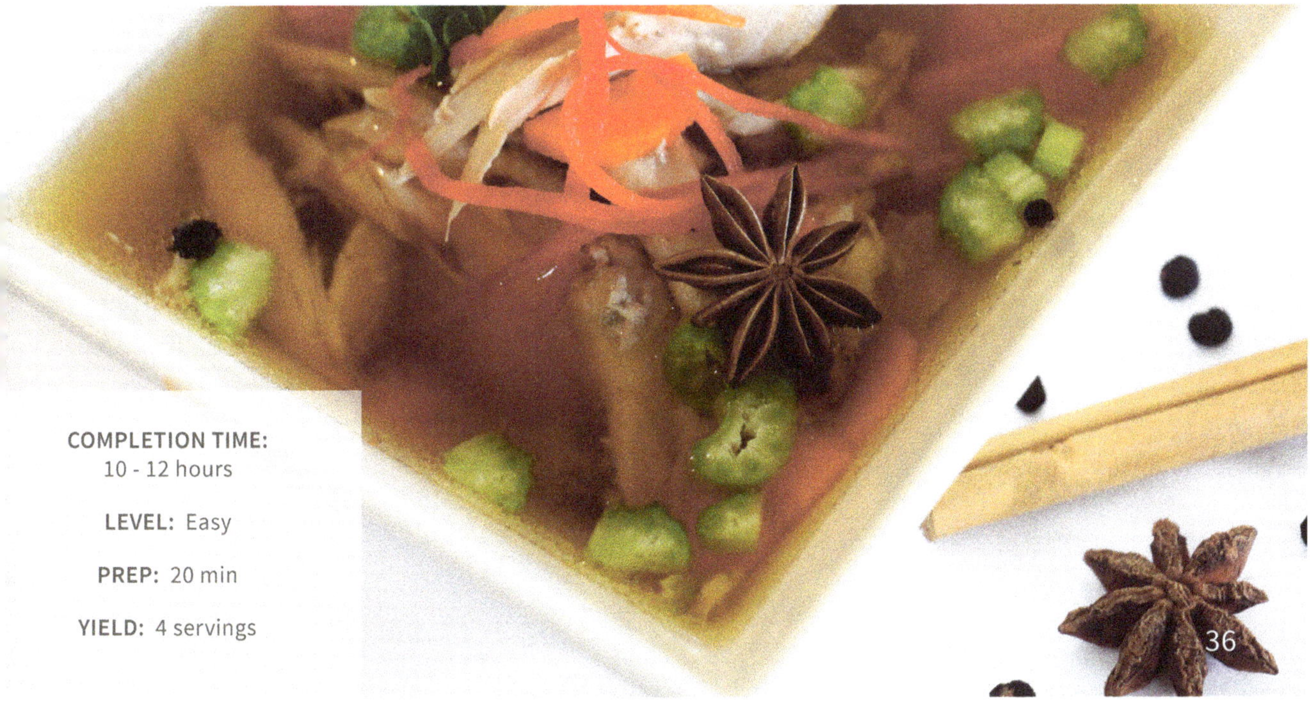

COMPLETION TIME: 10 - 12 hours

LEVEL: Easy

PREP: 20 min

YIELD: 4 servings

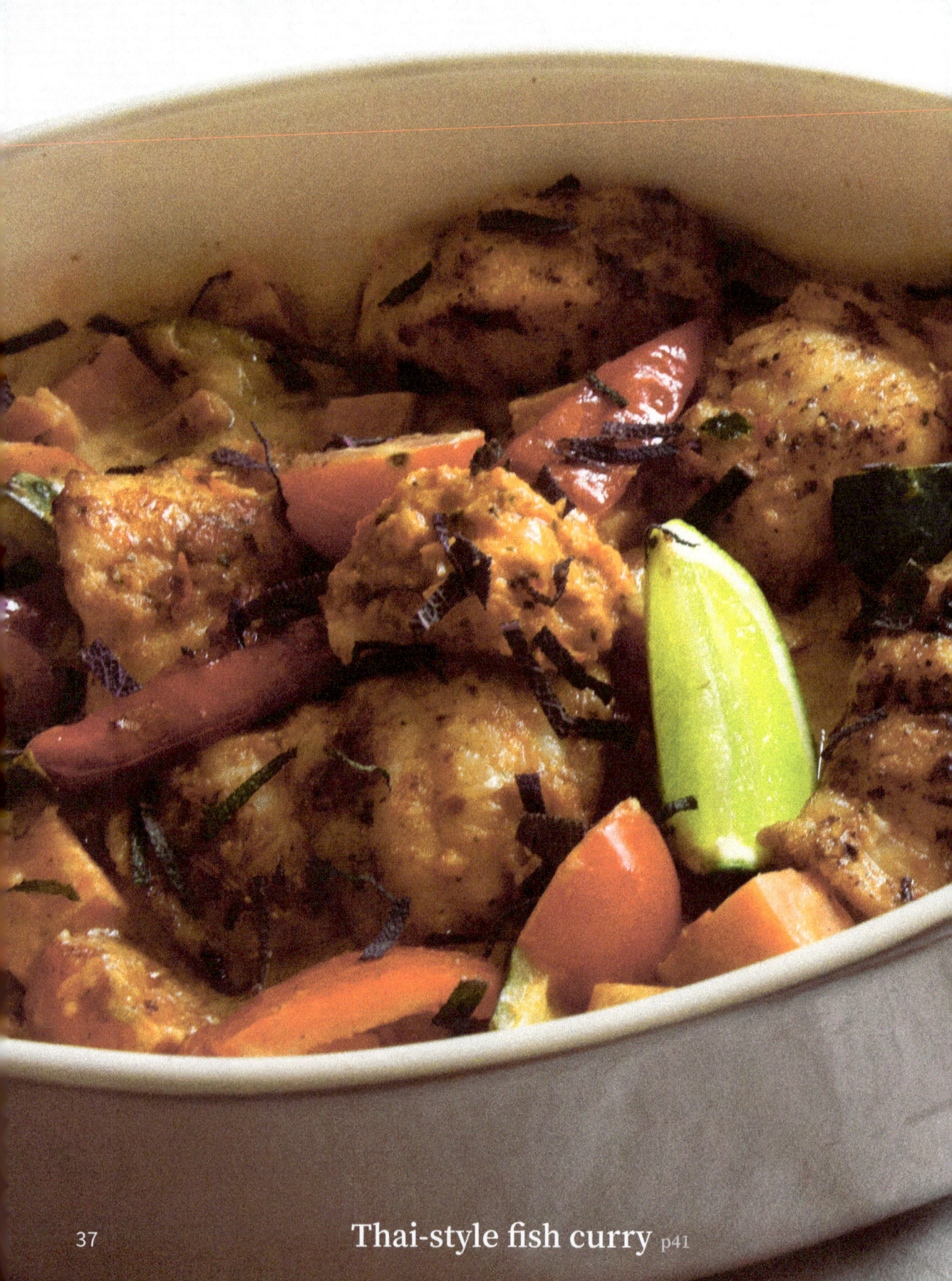

Thai-style fish curry p41

The Main Attraction
to share with the ones you love

Chicken stock & bone broths	40
Thai-style fish curry	41
Italian style perch with lemon, anchovies, capers & rosemary	42
Lemongrass rice salad	43
Pork san choy bau	44
Sautéed pork with lemon caper sauce	45
Moussaka (plant based)	48
Root vegetables roasted with hazelnuts	49
Roast vegetable medley	50
Coconut poached chicken with lime	51
Spicy beef pilaf	52
Spiced roast duck	53
Pizza with olives, anchovies & mushrooms	54
Slow cooked French rillette	55
Pickled wild salmon	56

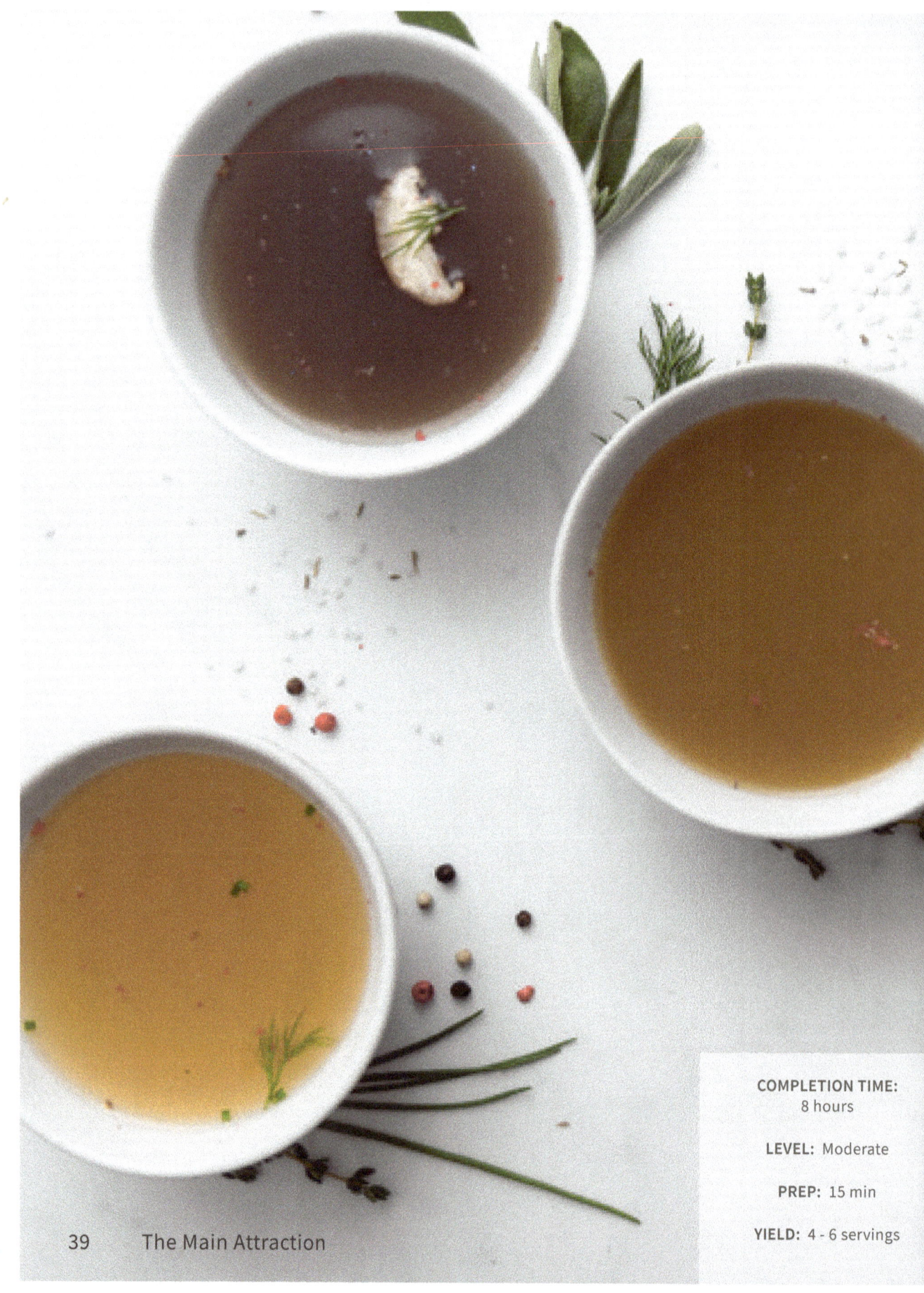

COMPLETION TIME: 8 hours

LEVEL: Moderate

PREP: 15 min

YIELD: 4 - 6 servings

Chicken stock & bone broths

Gluten Free Nut Free Dairy Free Sugar Free

Option: Use roasted bones of lamb or beef or pork to make a rich hearty stock.

Change your herbs to suit the meat for e.g. oregano to go with beef or rosemary with lamb, dill or ginger to go with fish frames, five spice, fennel and orange zest to go with pork.

Bone broth is made using meaty bones and is generally cooked for longer than a meat stock.

Ingredients

1 whole chicken cut into portions or 3 chicken frames

pure water to cover the meat

1 large carrot roughly chopped

2 sticks celery roughy chopped

1 large zucchini roughly chopped

1 tsp asafoetida

2 tsp dried porcini mushrooms

2 tsp dried or fresh sage leaf

6 peppercorns

salt to taste

Method

1. Place all of the ingredients into a large stock pot or slow cooker. Bring to the boil and reduce to a very slow simmer
2. Cook for around 6 hours until the meat falls easily from the bones
3. Allow to cool slightly
4. Using a slotted spoon lift the solids out into a bowl leaving the liquid behind
5. Option: boil the liquid rapidly to reduce to around 3 cups for easy storage in the fridge or reduce further to 1 cup to use as a sauce or flavour-packed addition to your *Not fast enough five minute casserole* (p60)

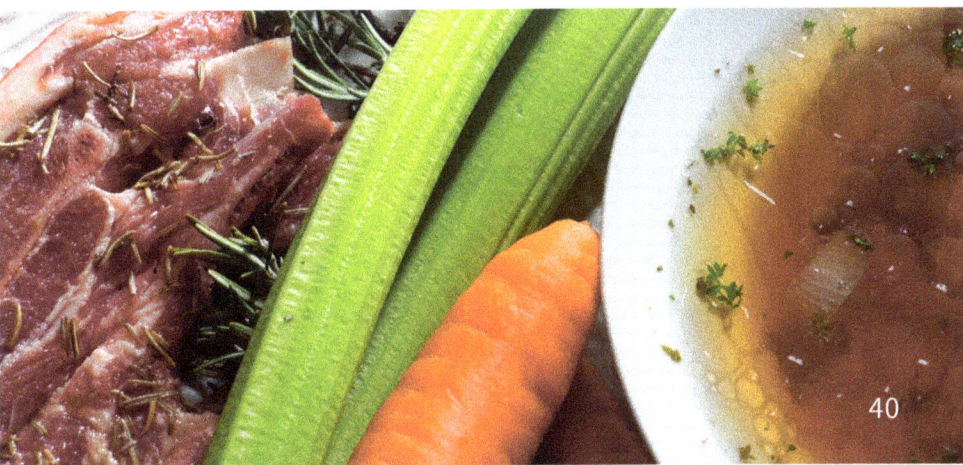

COMPLETION TIME: 60 min

LEVEL: Challenging

PREP: 45 min

YIELD: 6 servings

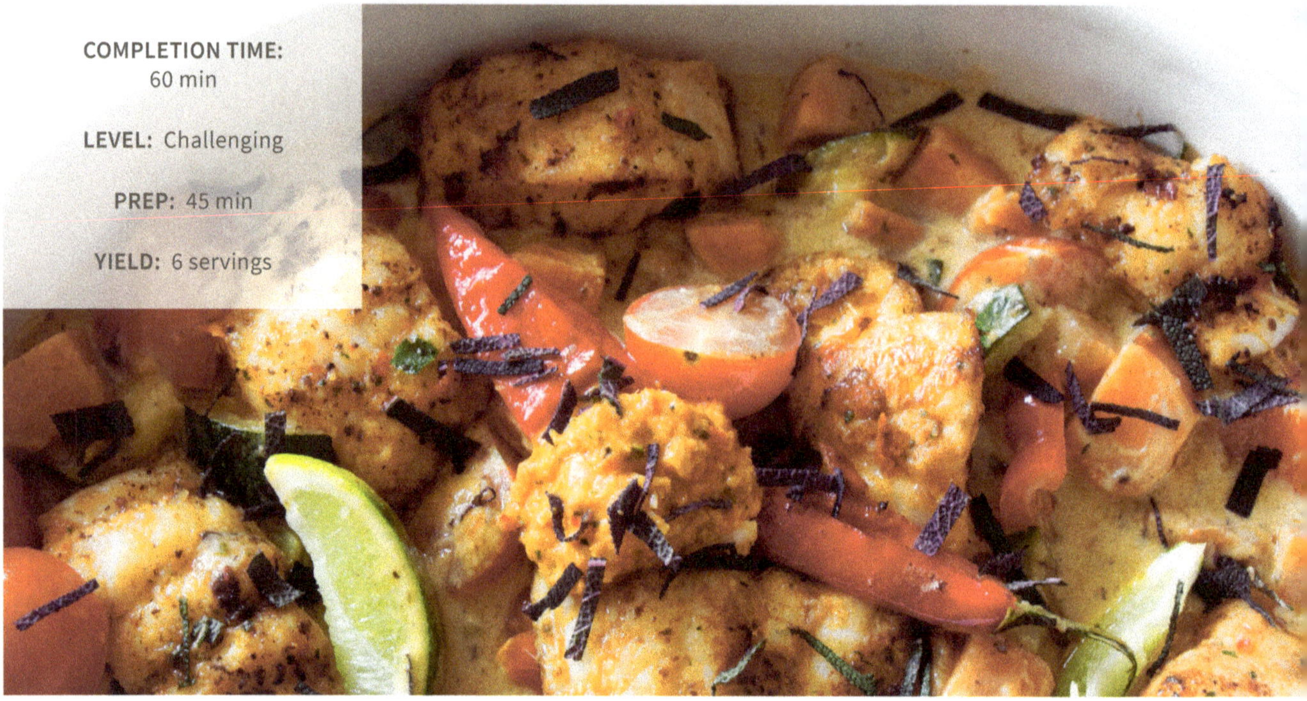

Thai-style fish curry

Gluten Free Nut Free Dairy Free Sugar Free

Avoid predatory fish which are known to contain high levels of mercury such as shark, ray, swordfish, barramundi, gemfish, orange roughy, ling, southern bluefin tuna. (These are southern hemisphere species- please refer to your local information resources). Look for smaller species whereby the whole fillet is not larger than a dinner plate.

Ingredients

750g of fresh fish fillets such as wild caught salmon, blue eye trevalla, flat head, flounder, snapper, mackerel
3 Tbs ghee
1 Tbs coconut oil
extra fresh Thai basil to Serve
cooked red rice to Serve
2 tsp fish sauce
1 lime sliced to serve
the juice of 1 lime
1 x 270ml can of coconut milk
2 tsp corn starch
1 red capsicum (pepper) cut into 2 cm squares
1/2 butternut or Jap pumpkin (squash) cut into 2 cm cubes
6 small potatoes cut in half
1 large zucchini (squash)
2 Tbs *Low thiol Thai curry paste* (p20)

Method

1. Cut the fish into 9 cm portions and marinate them in curry paste for 20 minutes
2. Heat half of the ghee and coconut oil together to a moderately-high heat in a large heavy-based fry pan
3. Place 2 Tbs of the curry paste and all of the vegetables into the pan and allow to brown lightly for 6 minutes, stir the vegetables around and continue to brown for another 6 minutes with a lid on the pan
4. Remove from the heat and stir through the fish sauce, coconut milk and lime juice
5. Set the vegetables aside in a casserole dish
6. Heat the remainder of the ghee and coconut oil in the same pan
7. Fry the fish in small batched (two to three pieces at a time) for around 2 minutes on each side until browned
8. Add the fish to the casserole dish, cover and place in a moderate oven for 30 minutes
9. Serve with rice and top with fresh basil leaves, slices of lime and cracked pepper

Italian style perch
with lemon, anchovies, capers & rosemary

Gluten Free   Nut Free   Dairy Free   Sugar Free

Ingredients

4 x 180g skinless ocean perch fillets
4 Tbs ghee
sea salt and freshly ground black pepper
2 large lemons finely sliced
2 Tbs of salted capers rinsed
1 tsp of fresh rosemary
8 anchovy fillets

Method

1. Preheat oven to 200°C or 400°F
2. Bruise rosemary in a pestle and mortar to bring out flavour
3. Warm the ghee in a small saucepan and add the rosemary
4. Put half of this mixture on and around the fish and season well with salt and pepper in an oven-proof baking dish
5. Lay 4 or 5 slices of lemon over each piece of fish
6. Sprinkle over capers and place anchovies over the top
7. Drizzle with remaining ghee mixture and bake for around 20 minutes
8. Rest and serve with your choice of salad or rice and vegetable

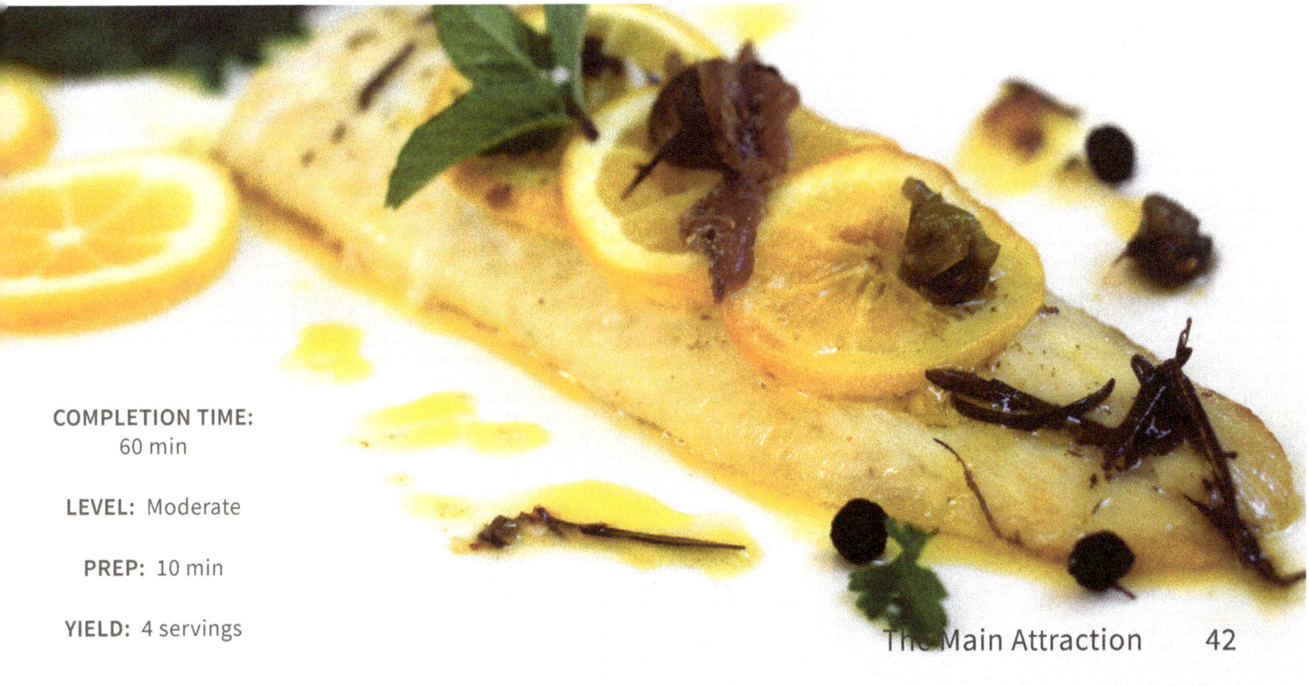

COMPLETION TIME: 60 min

LEVEL: Moderate

PREP: 10 min

YIELD: 4 servings

Lemongrass rice salad

Gluten Free   Nut Free   Dairy Free

Ingredients

2 Tbs coconut oil

2 stalks lemongrass sliced in half length-ways and each piece tied into a knot

3 red chillies, seeded and chopped

3 cups cooked rice (choose from red, wild or black rice or a combination. Jasmine works well)

2 cups cooked shredded or sliced chicken, pork, beef or lamb

1 cup shredded mint

1/2 cup shredded basil leaves

3 kaffir lime leaves finely shredded

3 Tbs lime juice

1 Tbs rapadura sugar

1 Tbs fish sauce

Method

1. Heat oil in frying pan and fry the lemongrass and chilli for 2 minutes to release the flavour
2. Into a bowl place the cooked rice, meat, mint, basil, lime leaves and lemongrass mixture and toss to combine
3. Mix the lime juice, sugar and fish sauce and add to the rice
4. Toss to combine and serve

Note: For vegetarian/vegan option leave out the chicken, pork, beef or lamb

COMPLETION TIME: 30 min

LEVEL: Moderate

PREP: 40 min

YIELD: 4 servings

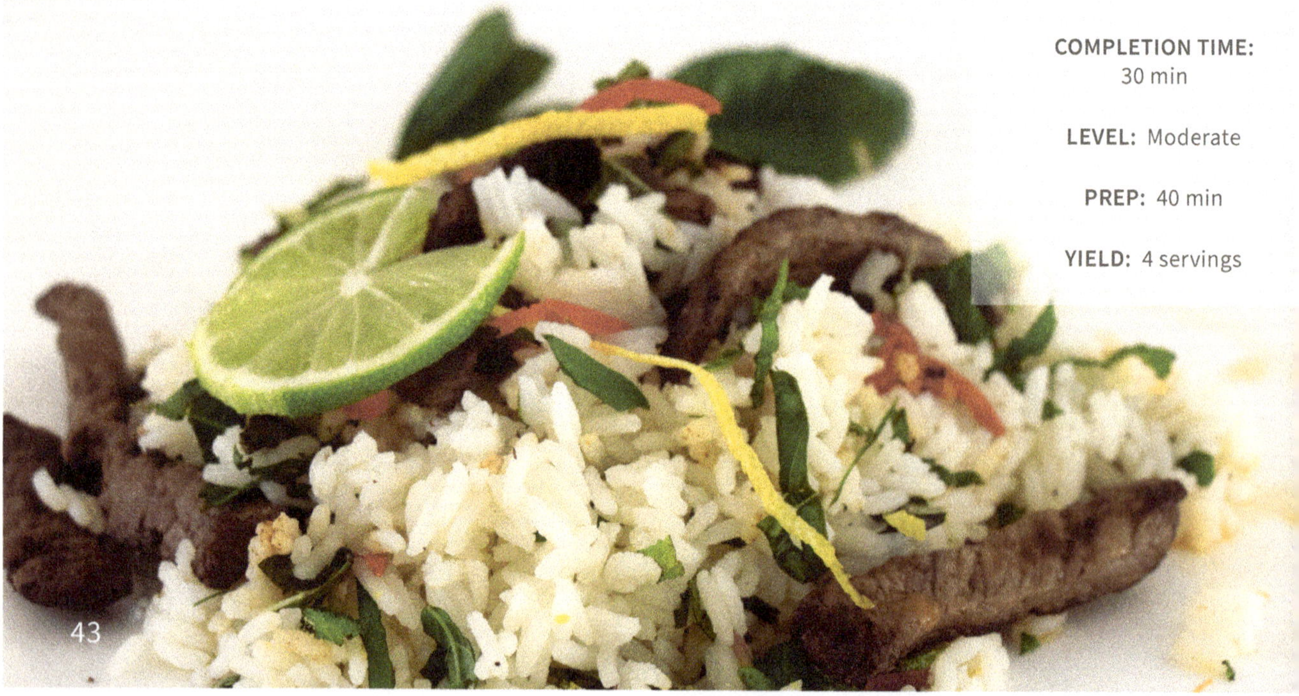

COMPLETION TIME: 30 min

LEVEL: Moderate

PREP: 1 day

YIELD: 2 - 4 servings

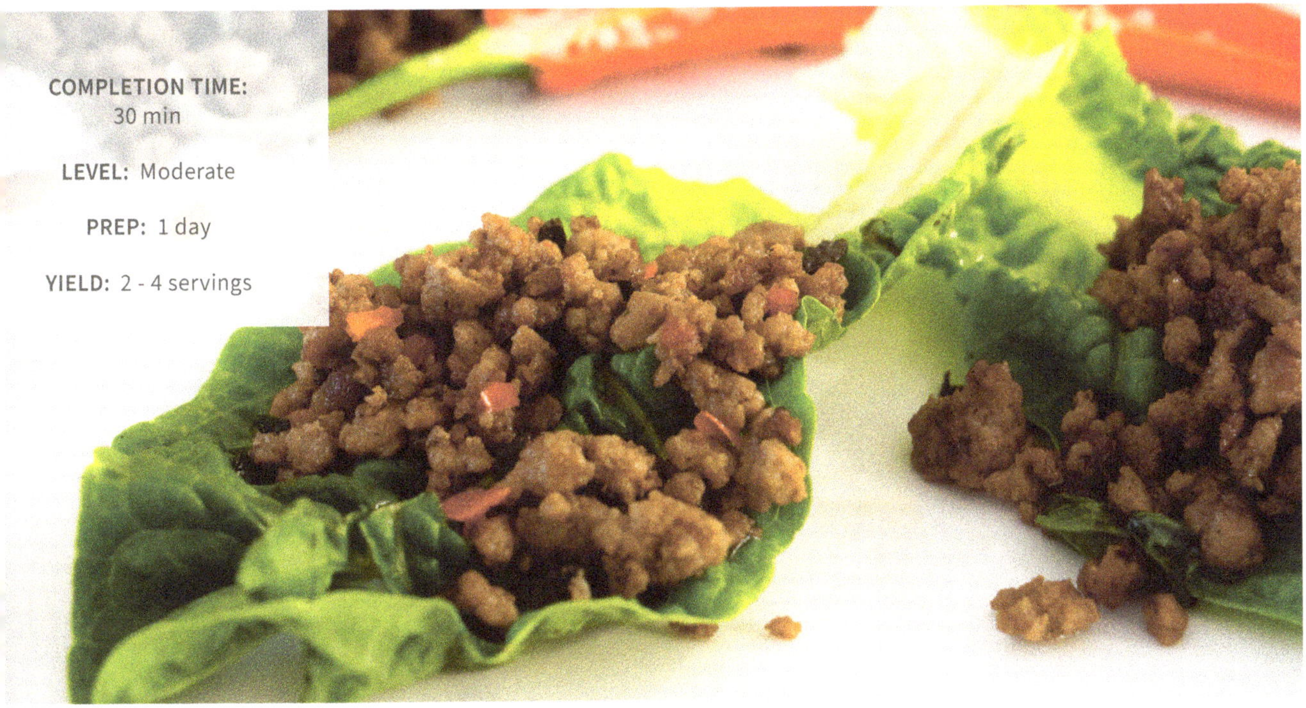

Pork san choy bau

Gluten Free · Nut Free · Dairy Free · Sugar Free

Fresh uncured pork can have an inflammatory effect for some individuals causing fatigue and bran fog. Marinating it in an acid together with salt and consuming with fermented vegetables helps to negate this effect.

Ingredients

200g free-range pork mince

1 Tbs of vinegar - choose from elderberry, rice or white wine vinegar

1 chilli finely diced

1 Tbs ghee

1/2 tsp five spice

1 1/2 Tbs fish sauce

2 Tbs lemon juice

2 Tbs coconut aminos

1 Tbs sesame oil

1/4 cup Thai basil leaves chopped

1/4 cup mint leaves chopped

baby cos lettuce leaves to serve

Method

1. In a bowl mix the vinegar, pork mince and fish sauce together with a fork. Allow to sit for several hours or overnight in the fridge
2. Heat the ghee in a heavy based fry pan
3. Fry pork mince on a high heat until golden brown
4. Add 5 spice and chilli and stir
5. Add lemon juice and coconut aminos and cook until liquid is reduced but not dry
6. Remove from heat and stir through sesame oil, Thai basil and mint leaves
7. Spoon into lettuce cups and serve with low thiol *Fermented vegetables* (p24)

The Main Attraction   44

Sautéed pork with lemon caper sauce

Gluten Free — Nut Free — Dairy Free — Sugar Free

Ingredients

Wrapper

4 boneless and skinless pork chops *pre-marinated. Ask the butcher to slice them as thinly as possible

1/4 cup cassava powder (or tapioca flour)

large pinch salt

3 Tbs ghee or duck fat for sautéing

Lemon Caper Sauce

3 Tbs rinsed capers

1/2 cup dry white wine

1/2 cup chicken stock *(p40)*

1 medium lemon

1 tsp cassava powder

1 Tbs fresh chopped parsley

Cassava powder is made from the Yucca root and is an excellent source of fibrous food for your gut bugs. **See our resource section.**

*Marinating fresh pork may reduce its inflammatory effects.
*Soak pork for 24 hours in enough pure water to cover mixed with 1 Tbs salt and 1 Tbs vinegar per 500ml of water. Rinse and pat dry before use.

Method

1. Preheat oven to 110°C or 230°F and place a baking tray in the oven to keep warm
2. If you are using pork chops that are thick, cut them in half lengthways to make them approximately 1 cm thick
3. Place each pork chop between two pieces of parchment paper and use a meat tenderiser to pound them into pieces approximately 1/2 cm thick
4. Mix the cassava flour and salt in a wide flat bowl and dip each piece of pork into the seasoned flour to coat evenly. Shake off any excess flour and transfer to a plate
5. Heat a large frying pan or sauté pan over a medium heat and add half of the ghee or oil
6. Cook the pork pieces in batches for a couple of minutes on each side until golden brown
7. Transfer the cooked pork to the oven to keep warm. Keep used pan for the sauce

Lemon Caper Sauce

8. Add the capers to the same pan, cook for a minute and add the white wine, half of the chicken stock and the lemon juice, stir with a wooden spoon to loosen up the browned pieces from the bottom of the pan
9. Simmer gently for a couple of minutes until the sauce thickens
10. In a small bowl or cup mix a teaspoon of cassava flour with a small amount of cold water and whisk
11. Add this mixture to the pan and stir constantly until the sauce is smooth
12. Add the remaining half of the chicken stock to the pan to thin the sauce a little
13. Taste and add an extra pinch of salt or lemon juice if needed
14. Stir in the parsley and remove from the heat
15. Serve the sauce poured over the cooked pork pieces

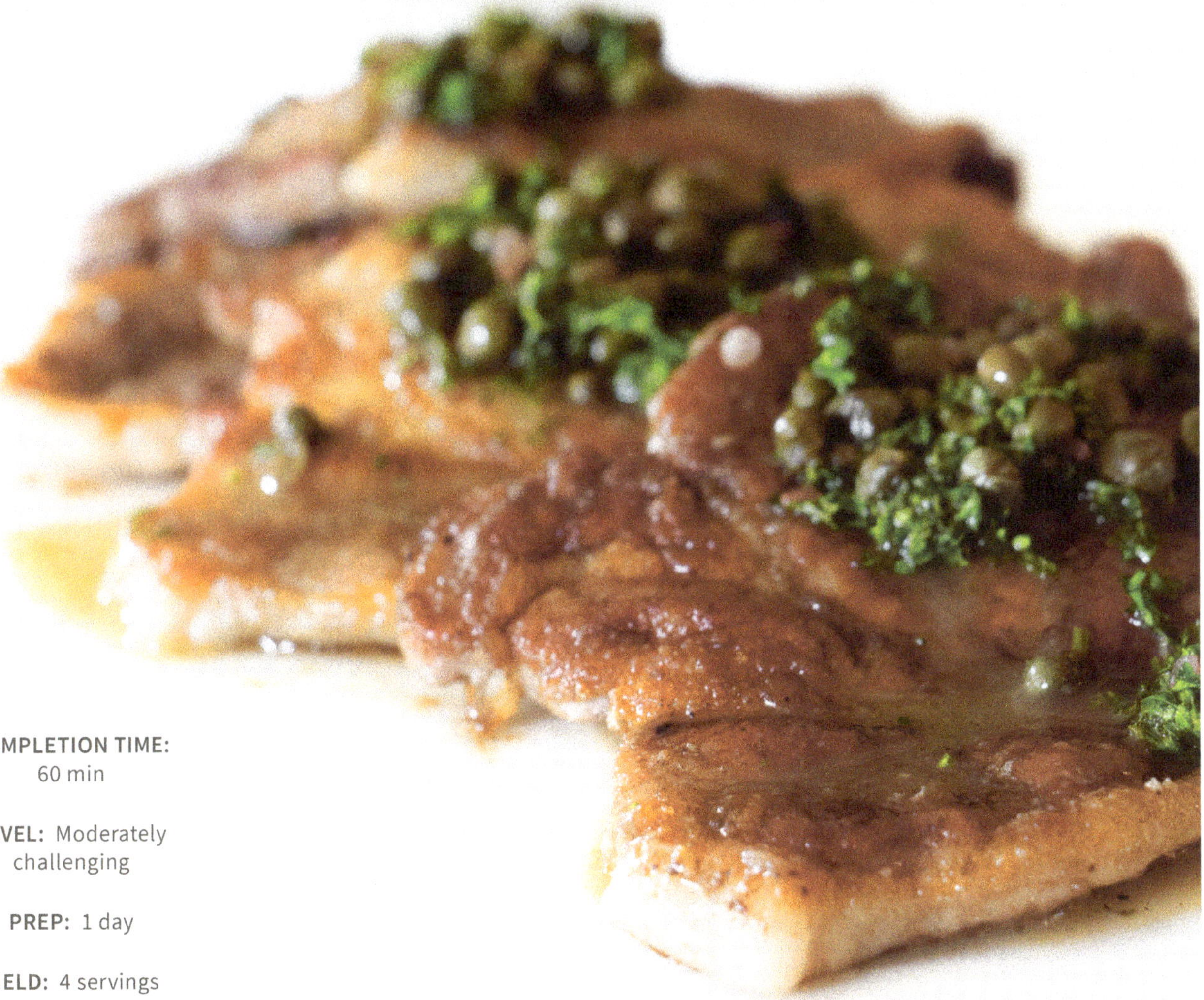

COMPLETION TIME:
60 min

LEVEL: Moderately challenging

PREP: 1 day

YIELD: 4 servings

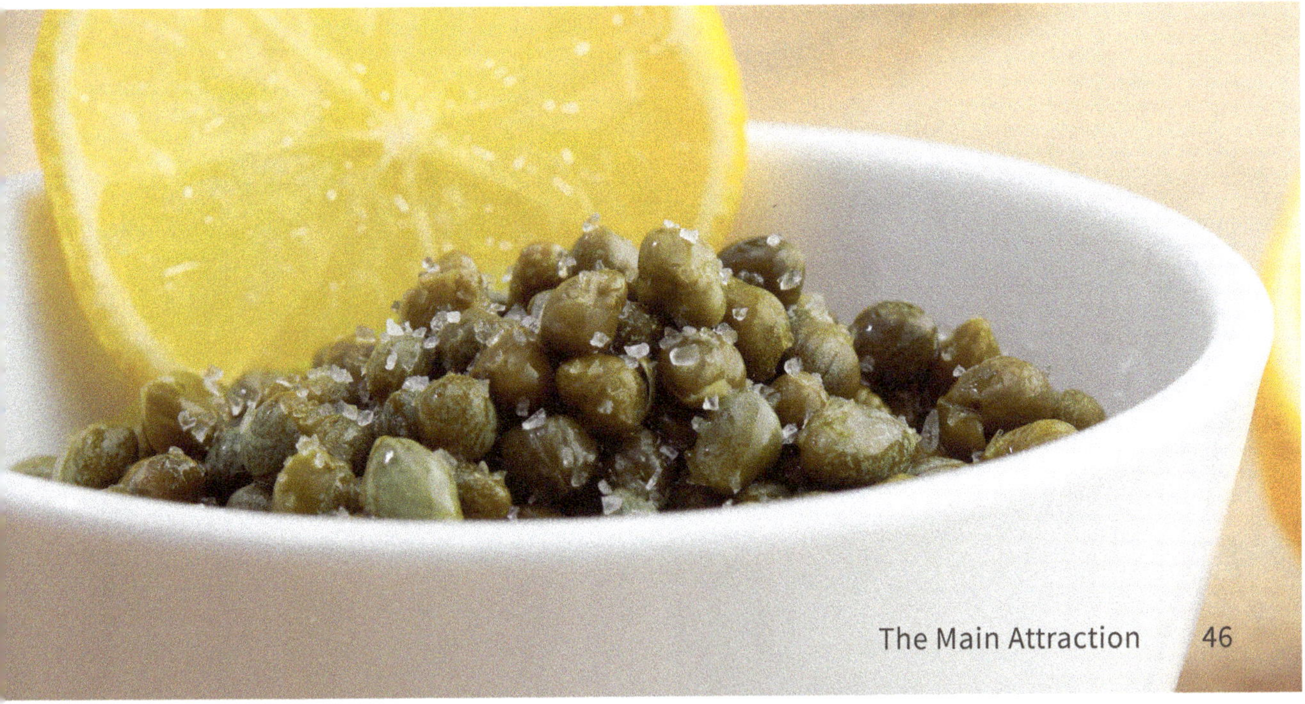

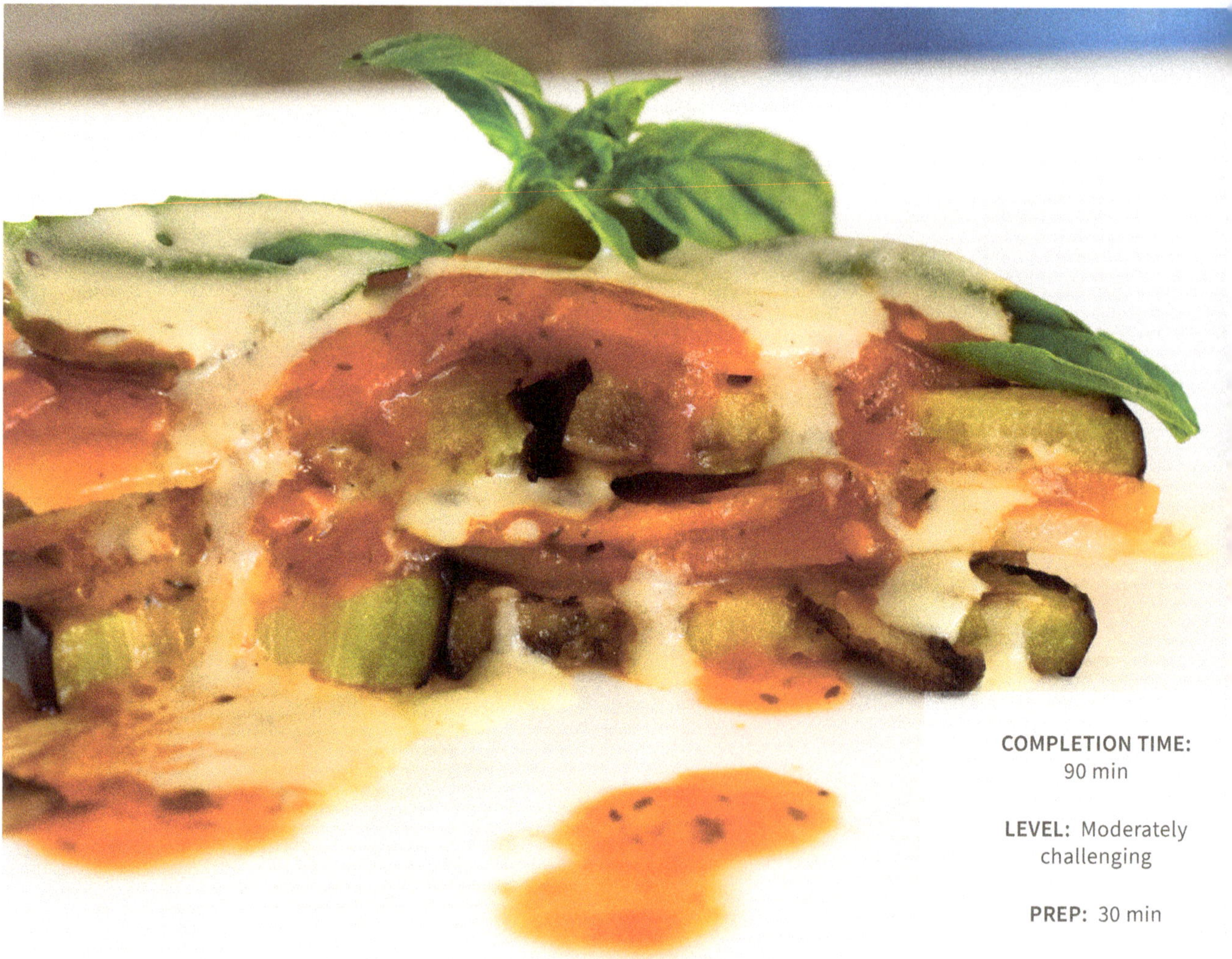

COMPLETION TIME:
90 min

LEVEL: Moderately challenging

PREP: 30 min

YIELD: 4 servings

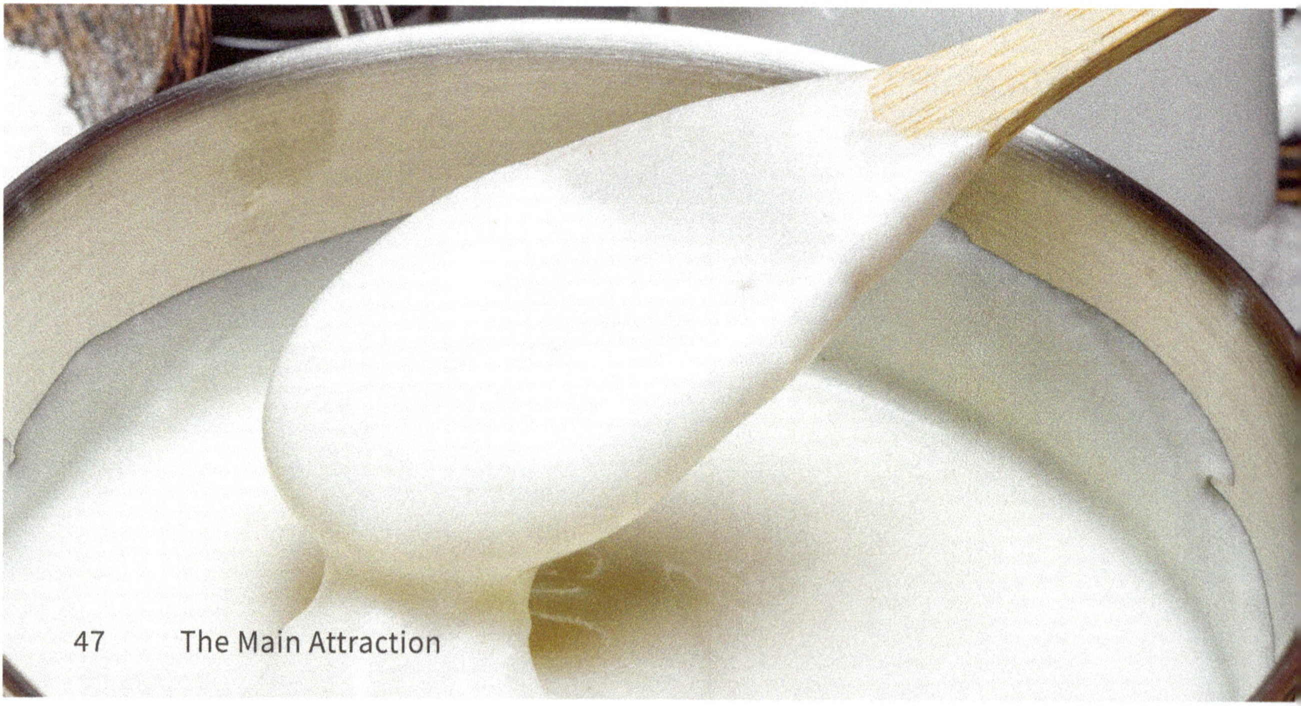

The Main Attraction

Moussaka (plant based)

Ingredients

2 Tbs olive oil
2 carrots sliced thinly
1 eggplant sliced thinly
2 large floury potatoes sliced
2 tomatoes, chopped
1 cup sliced mushrooms
2 bay leaves
1 Tbs thyme leaves
800g of diced tomatoes (bottled)
1 cup vegetable stock *(p16)*
salt to taste

Note: Opt for fresh or tomatoes in glass as opposed to tinned tomatoes. The acid in the tomatoes causes leaching of the metals from the tin.

Method

1. Preheat oven to 220°C or 390°F
2. Heat oil in a large frying pan over medium heat, sauté small batches of the carrot, eggplant, potato, fresh tomatoes, and mushrooms until almost tender
3. Set aside in a bowl
4. Add the bay leaves and thyme, chopped tomatoes and stock to the same frying pan, season and bring to the boil
5. Cook for a further 2 minutes

Assemble

6. Arrange layers of the cooked vegetables, tomato sauce and Béchamel in a 2.5 litre oven-proof baking dish and top with the béchamel sauce and chopped parsley
7. Bake the moussaka for 45 minutes or until bubbling and slightly brown on top. Serve with extra parsley and basil

Béchamel Sauce

Ingredients

2 1/2 cups coconut milk (nut-free option) or activated* almond milk
2 Tbsp organic tapioca starch
1/2 tsp salt
1/8 tsp ground nutmeg
basil leaves and parsley to garnish

Method

1. Add 1/2 cup almond milk to medium saucepan
2. Mix in the tapioca starch, salt and nutmeg
3. Whisk until all ingredients are well combine and add the remaining milk
4. Stir constantly over a medium heat until the mixture thickens
5. Remove from the heat

*For more information about why it is important to activate nuts, see page xxiv

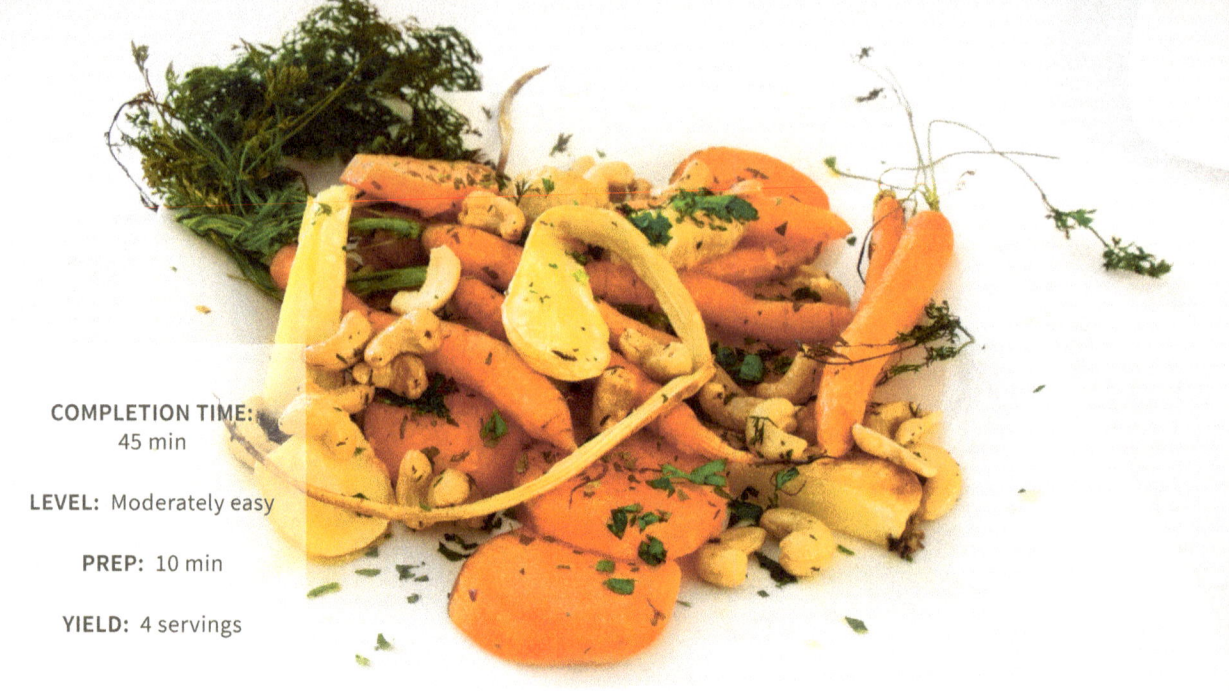

COMPLETION TIME: 45 min

LEVEL: Moderately easy

PREP: 10 min

YIELD: 4 servings

Root vegetables roasted with hazelnuts

Ingredients

1 Tbs melted ghee
4 carrots sliced lengthways
4 parsnips sliced lengthways
1 medium sweet potato diced
1 large yam or red skinned potato diced
1/3 cup activated* hazelnuts
2 Tbs hazelnut oil
1/4 cup chopped parsley
salt and pepper to taste

Variation: brazil nuts or cashews may be substituted for the hazelnuts.

Method

1. Place carrots, parsnips, sweet potato and yam into a baking pan and combine with the melted ghee
2. Roast on medium to high heat for about 30 minutes. Remove from oven and toss through the hazelnuts
3. Return to oven and roast for a further 30 minutes or until the vegetables are tender and golden
4. Drizzle with hazelnut oil and sprinkle with chopped parsley, salt and pepper
5. Serve warm or at room temperature

*For more information about why it is important to activate nuts, see page xxiv

Roast vegetable medley

Gluten Free   Nut Free   Vegetarian   Dairy Free   Sugar Free

Prepare an extra tray of vegetables to have on hand for soup or salads. Refer to our "I'm just too tired" recipe section (p57).

Ingredients

4 Tbs melted ghee

2 sprigs of rosemary

1 large eggplant cut into chunks

3 zucchini sliced

2 cups of butternut pumpkin (squash) diced

1 cup sliced red and green capsicum (peppers)

2 parsnip sliced lengthwise

6 whole baby carrot with tops left on

1 Tbs of fresh thyme

Method

1. Heat the oven to 180°C or 350°F fan forced
2. Rinse the vegetables
3. Place all of the vegetables and herbs apart from a sprig of thyme into a baking tray and drizzle with melted ghee
4. Roast for approximately 45 minutes or until vegetables are tender
5. Remove from oven and toss through thyme, salt and pepper
6. Serve warn or at room temperature

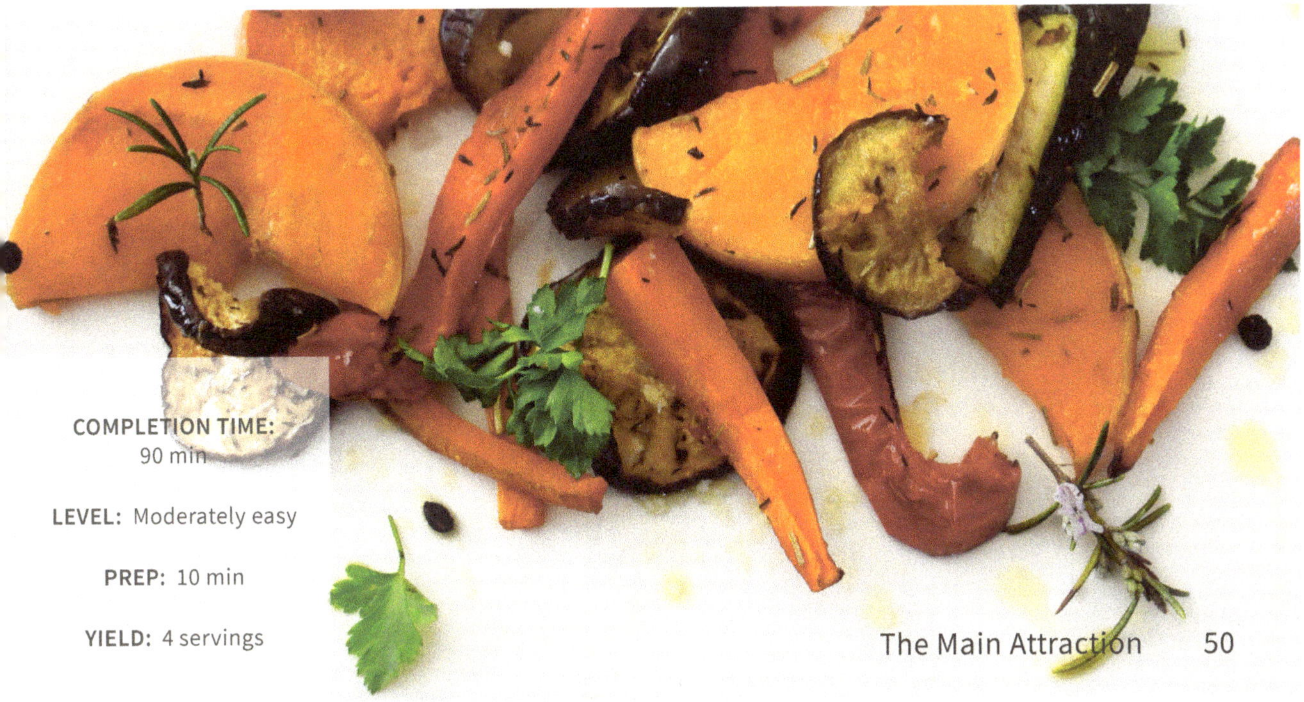

COMPLETION TIME: 90 min

LEVEL: Moderately easy

PREP: 10 min

YIELD: 4 servings

The Main Attraction

COMPLETION TIME: 60 min

LEVEL: Moderate

PREP: 15 min

YIELD: 4 servings

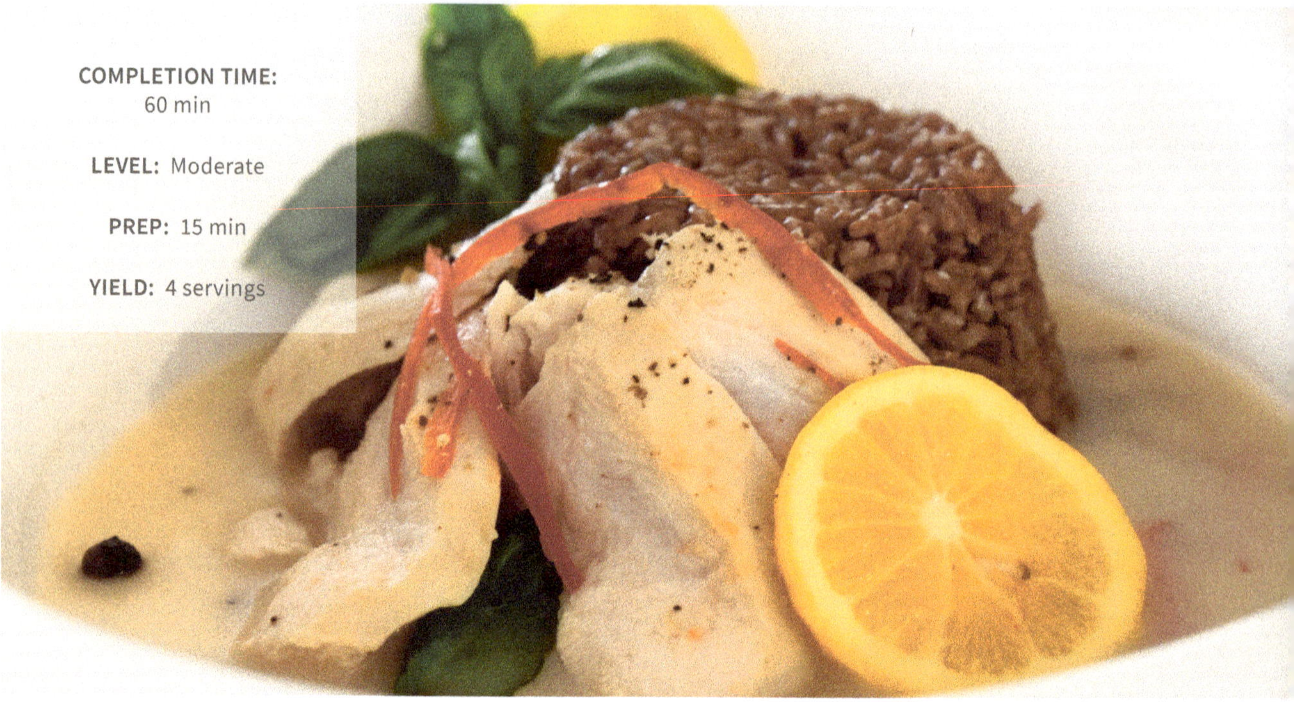

Coconut poached chicken with lime

Gluten Free Nut Free Dairy Free Sugar Free

Ingredients

1 litre chicken stock *(p40)*
1 can of coconut milk
1 lime or lemon
1 chilli
2 cm piece of ginger
2 boneless skinless organic chicken breasts
salt and pepper

Method

1. Combine chicken stock and coconut milk in a large saucepan over a low heat, DO NOT boil
2. Slice lime or lemon and chilli and add to poaching liquid
3. Peel and thinly slice ginger and add to poaching liquid with salt and pepper
4. Add chicken breast to the poaching liquid and bring heat up to a gentle simmer
5. Simmer the chicken for about 20 minutes
6. Remove chicken from liquid and keep warm
7. Reduce the liquid by rapidly boiling uncovered pan until there is around 1/2 cup of liquid
8. Serve with rice and steamed vegetables
9. Pour the stock reduction over the chicken

If like me you prefer skin-on chicken pieces you can pan sear the pieces skin down in a hot pan before adding to the poaching liquid. The skin provides collagen which is beneficial for gut, skin and joint health.

COMPLETION TIME: 40 min

LEVEL: Moderate

PREP: 40 min

YIELD: 4 servings

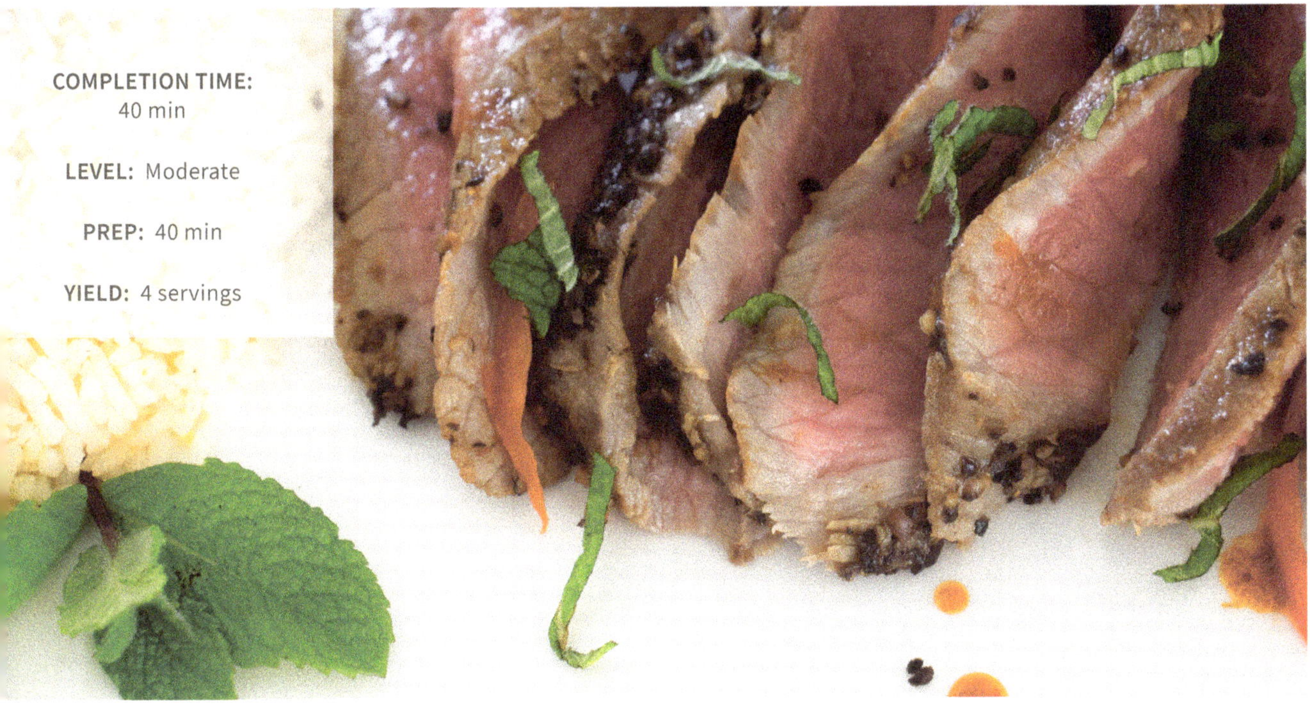

Spicy beef pilaf

 Gluten Free   Nut Free   Dairy Free   Sugar Free

Ingredients

2 cups basmati rice which has been well rinsed in a sieve
3 1/2 cups lamb or beef stock *(p40)*
2 cinnamon sticks
3 green cardamom pods, crushed
5 saffron threads
4 pieces of beef fillet or sirloin steak
1 1/2 Tbs chilli paste (below)
chopped mint (optional)

Chilli Paste

4 fresh red chillies
1/2 tsp salt
1 tsp ground cumin
1 tsp ground fennel seeds
1 Tbs olive oil
Himalayan salt and pepper to taste
1 Tbs ghee

Method

1. Make the chilli paste- halve the chillies and discard the seeds, finely chop. Combine the chillies, salt, pepper, cumin, fennel and oil using a mortar and pestle to form a smooth paste. Spread a small amount of chilli paste onto each portion of beef and set aside

2. Place washed rice, stock, cinnamon, cardamom and saffron into a large saucepan ensuring that the liquid is 1 1/2 cm above the rice. Bring to the boil. Cover with a tight fitting lid and reduce heat to a low setting. Cook the rice for 12 minutes or until tender.

3. Remove the cinnamon and cardamom pods

4. Gently sauté the remaining chilli paste in half the ghee and stir through the cooked rice. Keep the rice warm in a covered serving dish

5. Heat the remaining ghee and cook the pieces of beef over a high heat for 5 minutes each side for a 'medium' result. Allow the beef to rest for a couple of minutes and slice

6. Serve rice onto plates and top with the beef pieces, sprinkle with chopped mint

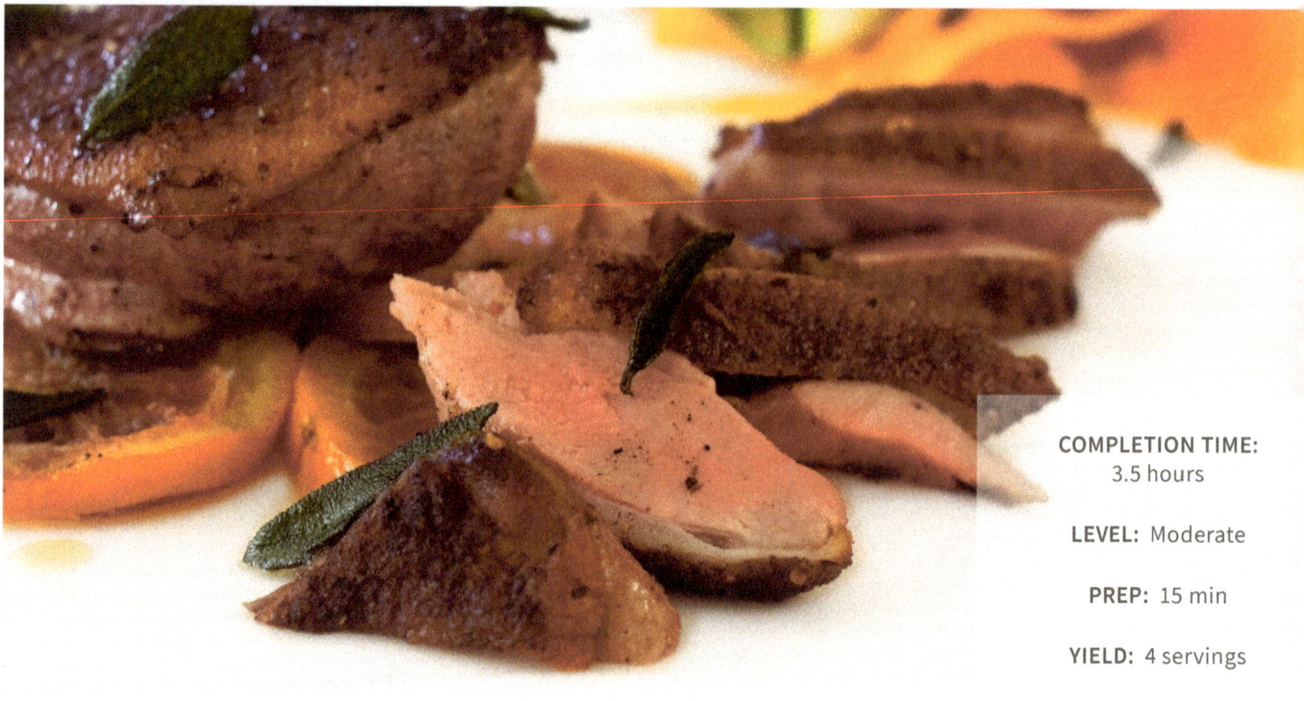

COMPLETION TIME: 3.5 hours

LEVEL: Moderate

PREP: 15 min

YIELD: 4 servings

Spiced roast duck

Gluten Free   Nut Free   Dairy Free

Option: Duck is commonly cooked 'confit' to produce a tender, moist meat with a crispy skin. Cut the raw duck into portions, rub with the seasonings and brown the skin in a hot pan. Place the portions into a deep oven dish and cover with duck fat before cooking at 110°C for around 3 1/2 hours.

Ingredients

1 duck, giblets removed
1 orange cut in half
3 sprigs fresh sage
2 Tbs *Jillaine's savoury ground spice blend (p99)*
salt and pepper

Dressing

2 fresh chillies
2 Tbs sesame oil
2 Tbs lime juice
1 tsp rapadura sugar

Method

1. Preheat oven to 180°C or 350°F
2. Wash the duck inside and out and pat dry with a clean cloth or kitchen paper
3. Place in a roasting tray and stuff with the orange halves and sprigs of sage
4. Mix the five spice powder with the salt and pepper and rub all over the duck
5. Turn the duck breast down into the pan and roast in the oven for about an hour
6. Remove the tray from the oven and spoon or pour all of the duck fat out of the tray through a sieve and into a heatproof bowl. Allow to cool
7. Turn the duck over and return to the oven to roast for a further 2 hours
8. After 2 hours, remove the tray from the oven and again spoon or pour the fat out of the tray and into the bowl
9. Cut the duck into portions and serve with dressing

DRESSING

1. Combine chillies, sesame oil and lime juice and sugar together and pour over the hot duck portions

Pizza with olives, anchovies & mushrooms

 Gluten Free   Nut Free   Vegetarian   Dairy Free   Sugar Free

Ingredients

2 cups roasted and mashed sweet potatoes

3/4 cup coconut flour

1/4 cup tapioca starch or arrowroot

salt and pepper

1 Tbs spices or herbs of choice

1 cup pureed roasted tomatoes

1 Tbs thyme leaves

12 olives pitted and halved

12 anchovies

1 cup sliced mushrooms

ghee or olive oil from anchovy jar for basting

Method

1. Combine sweet potatoes, coconut flour, tapioca starch, salt, pepper and herbs
2. In a mixing bowl. Mix to form 4 equal sized balls. Roll or pat each ball to about 1 cm thickness
3. Cook each base in a non stick pan for 5 minutes each side over a medium heat. When the base no longer sticks to the bottom of the pan it is ready to turn
4. Baste the top of each base with ghee or olive oil from anchovies
5. Top each base with a little tomato sauce and add the olives, anchovies, mushrooms and thyme leaves
6. Bake in a hot oven or pizza oven until the crusts are golden, about 10 - 15 minutes

Variation: 1 cup of shredded capsicum and 6 slices of roasted zucchini may be substituted for the olives and anchovies or, use any left over Roast vegetable medley (p50) as a topping.

COMPLETION TIME: 90 min

LEVEL: Moderately challenging

PREP: 40 min

YIELD: 4 servings

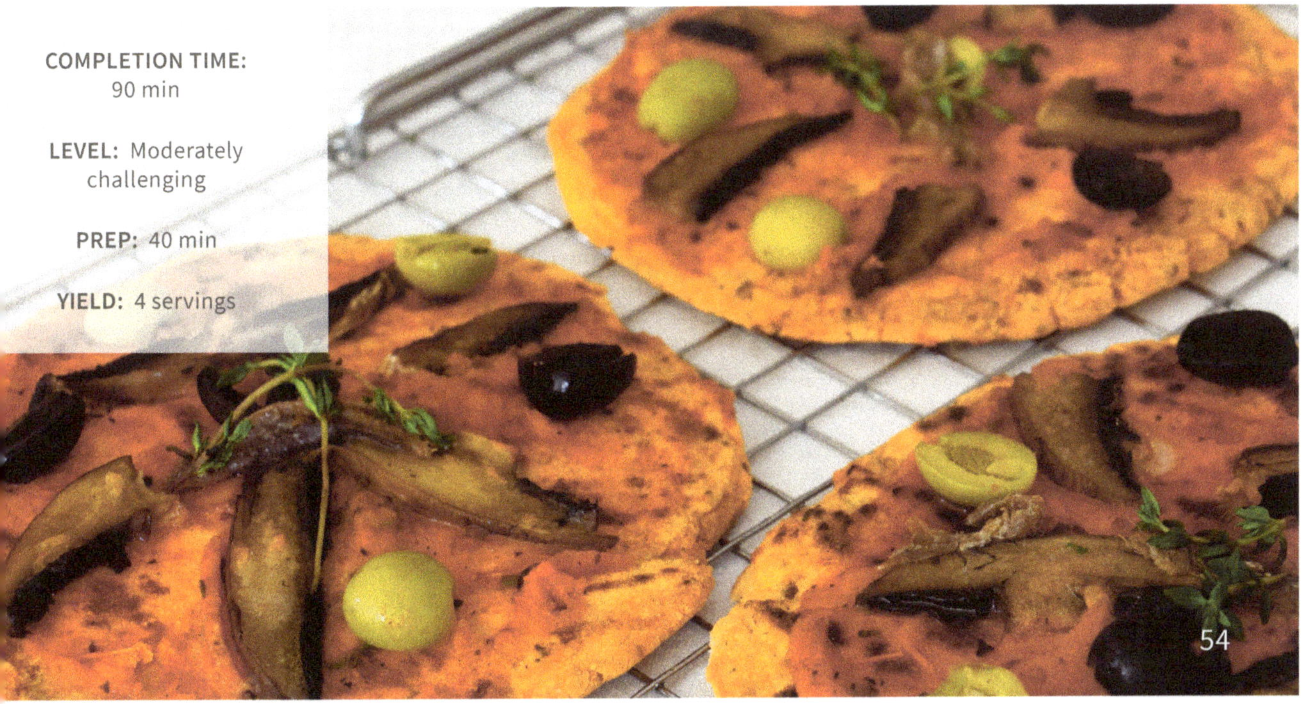

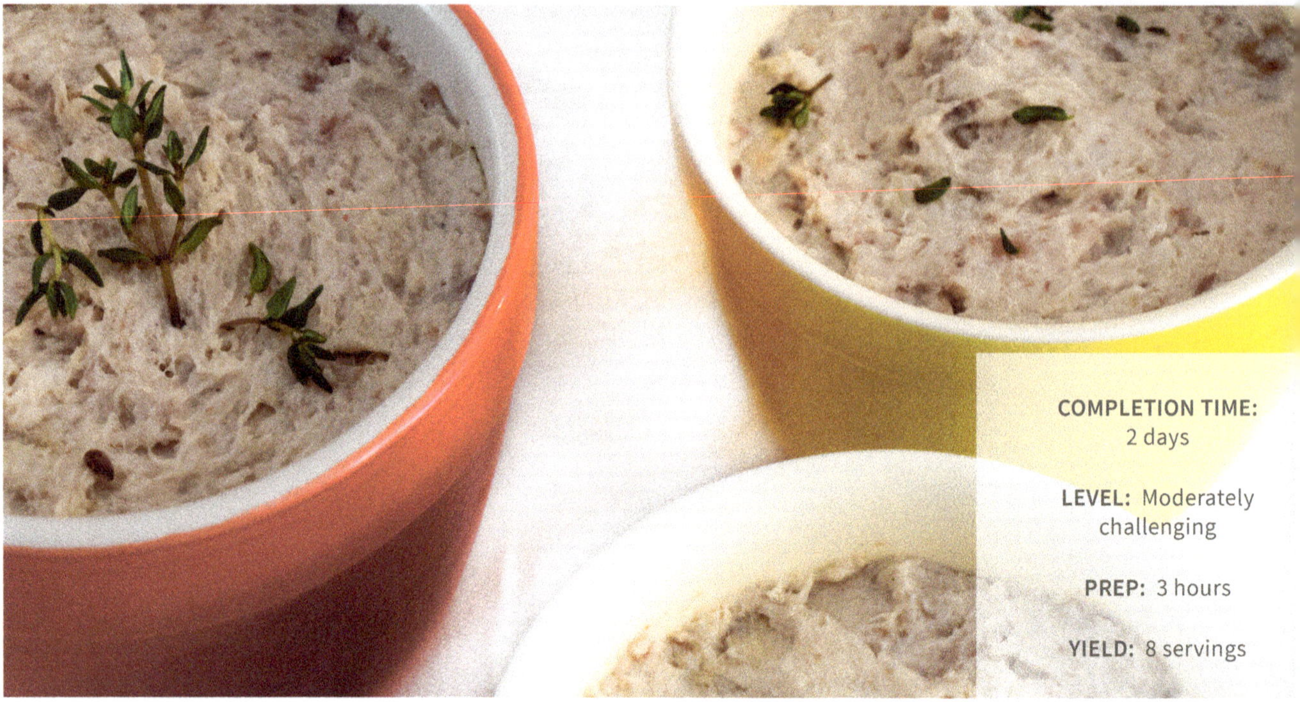

Slow cooked French rillette

 Gluten Free   Nut Free   Dairy Free   Sugar Free

COMPLETION TIME: 2 days

LEVEL: Moderately challenging

PREP: 3 hours

YIELD: 8 servings

Ingredients

1/2 kilo rindless, fatty pork belly cut into cubes *

1 rabbit or chicken jointed (cut into pieces on the bone)

4 bay leaves

1 sprig of fresh thyme

salt and pepper

1/4 tsp mixed spice

1/2 tsp allspice

shaved nutmeg

1/2 cup water

1/2 cup dry white wine

*Marinating fresh pork has been shown to reduce its inflammatory effects.

Soak pork for 24 hours in a brine made with enough pure water to cover mixed with 1 Tbs salt per 500ml water and 1 Tbs vinegar per 500ml of water. Rinse and pat dry before use.

Method

1. See slow cooker method below or place the meat pieces into a stainless roasting pan in a single layer
2. Add the bay leaves and thyme and pour over the wine and water
3. Roast at 220°C or 420°F for 30 minutes then turn down to 140°C or 280°F and cook for a further 2 1/2 to 3 hours until the meat is cooked through and tender
4. Remove from oven, allow to cool and pull the meat off the bones into a large bowl. Discard the bones
5. Shred the meats including the pork with 2 forks or use your hands
6. Place the roasting pan over a moderate flame or transfer the pan juices to a large saucepan. Add the spices and boil rapidly to reduce the liquid to around 1 cup
7. Pour the sauce over the meats and mix well ensuring the sauce is distributed throughout the meats evenly. Add at least a tsp of salt and cracked pepper to your taste
8. Transfer to ramekin bowls cover and refrigerator for a couple of days, this helps enhance the flavour
9. When completely chilled turn the Rillettes out onto a plate and serve with toast, salad greens and an olive oil and lemon dressing

Option: This recipe works well in a slow cooker for around 8 hours on the lowest setting. Continue as per recipe from step 6.

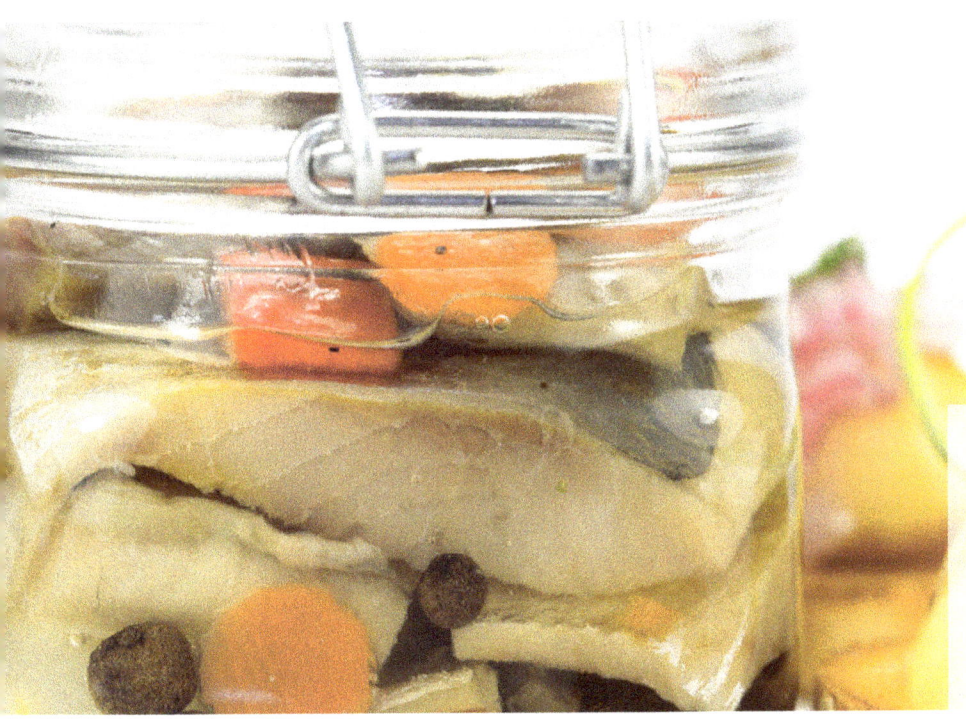

COMPLETION TIME: 24 hours

LEVEL: Moderate

PREP: 15 min

YIELD: 4 servings

Pickled wild salmon

 Gluten Free   Nut Free   Dairy Free   Sugar Free

Ingredients

1/2 kilo wild salmon or wild, local oily fish skinned and cut into 2 cm pieces

1 cup pure water

2 Tbs *Kombucha* (p93)

1 Tbs raw honey

1 Tbs sea salt

1 lemon thinly sliced

1 tsp cracked pepper

3 bay leaves

1 bunch fresh dill

Method

1. Mix water with Kombucha, honey and salt until salt and honey have dissolved. Stir in lemon slices, mustard seeds, pepper, bay leaves and dill and fish
2. Place into a large wide mouth jar
3. Ensure that the fish is covered with liquid, add more water if necessary
4. Cover jar tightly
5. Store at room temperature for 24 hours then place in the refrigerator

Pickled fish will keep for a number of weeks under refrigeration.

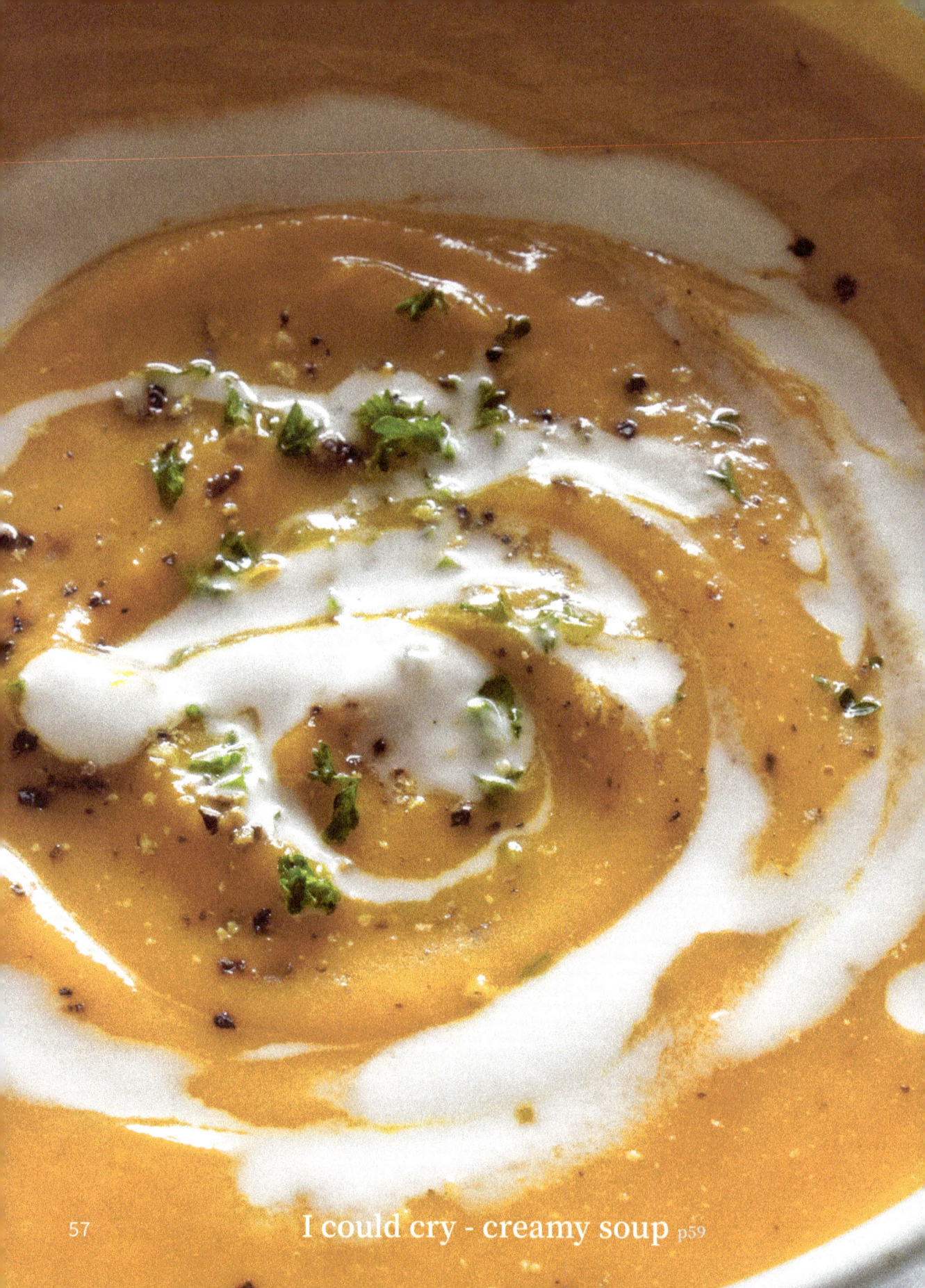
I could cry - creamy soup p59

I'm Just Too Tired To Cook!

quick easy solutions that warm the soul & nourish the body

I could cry - creamy soup	59	Right now roast	63
Not fast enough five minute casserole	60	Resuscitating Thai curry	64
Suddenly salad	62		

COMPLETION TIME:
5 min

LEVEL: Easy

PREP: 5 min

YIELD: 4 servings

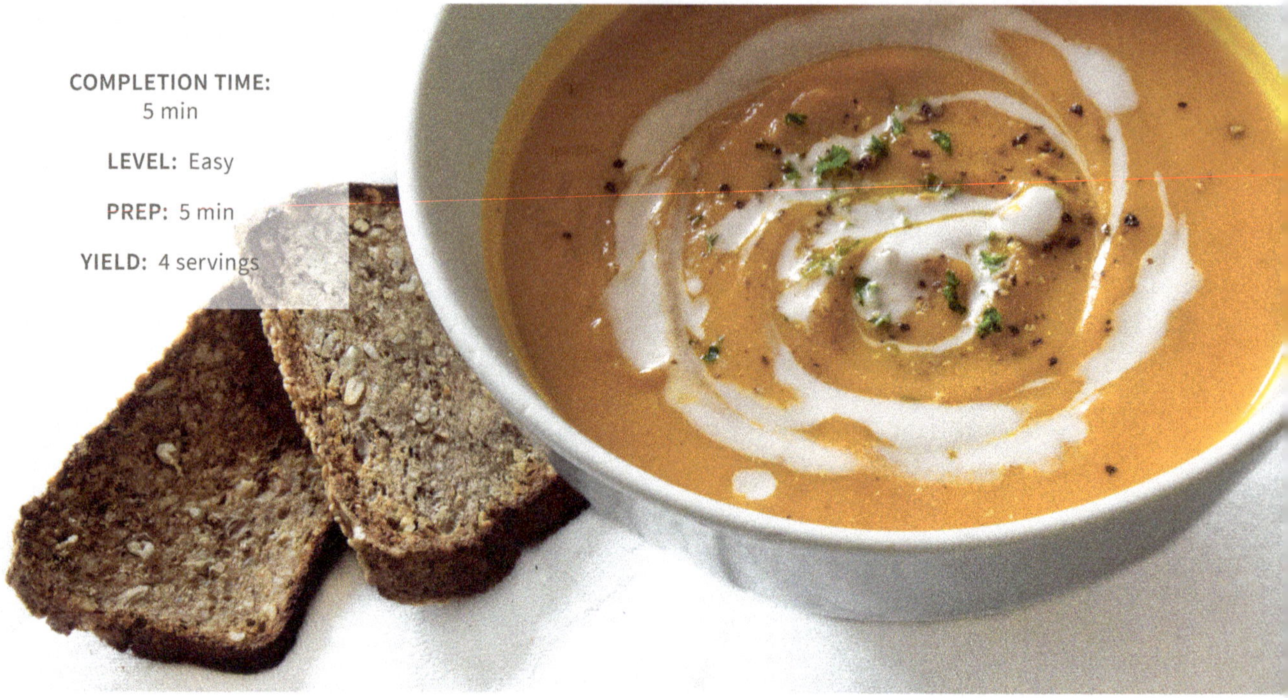

I could cry - creamy soup

Gluten Free · Nut Free · Vegetarian · Dairy Free · Sugar Free

Ingredients

left over roast vegetables

Meat stock *(p40)* or vegetable stock *(p16)*

salt and pepper to taste

coconut cream to serve (optional)

Method

1. Blend the vegetables with hot stock until smooth and cream
2. Top with salt and pepper and coconut cream

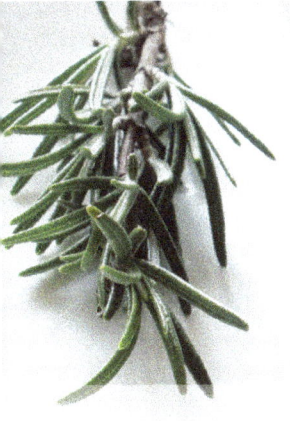
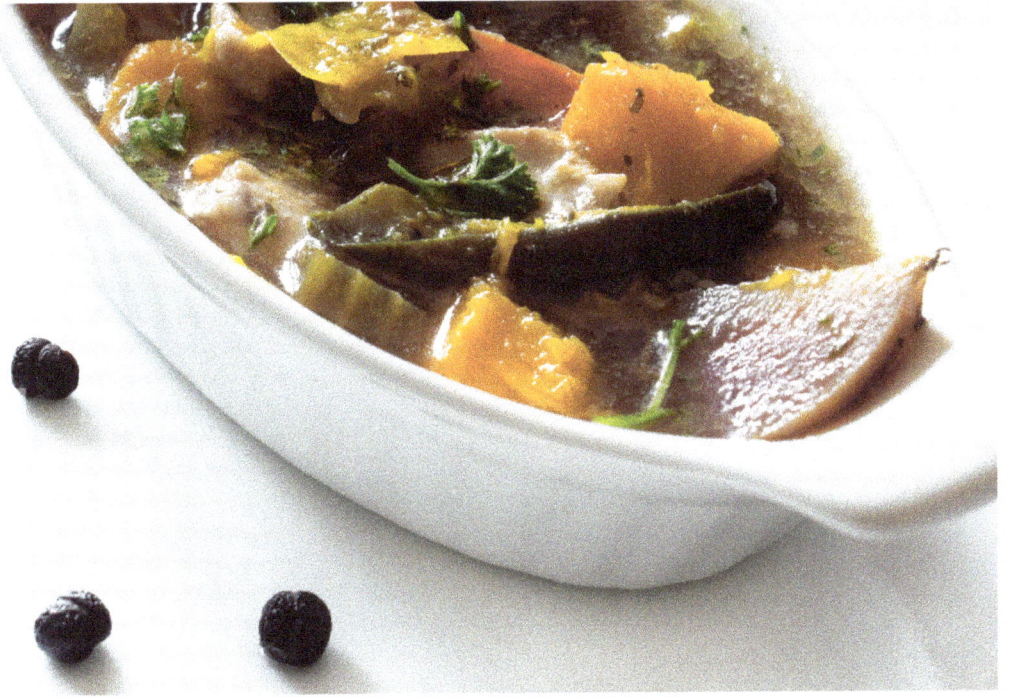

COMPLETION TIME: 3 min

LEVEL: Easy

PREP: 2 min

YIELD: 4 servings

Not fast enough five minute casserole

Ingredients

stock reduction

left over roasted vegetables

left over roast or slow cooked meat cut into cubes or shredded

extra ghee

salt and pepper to taste

chopped fresh herb of your choice

Method

1. Place the broth, meat and vegetables into a saucepan and warm through
2. Top with fresh herb salt and pepper
3. Serve with *Cumin flatbread* (p87) or gluten-free toast and ghee

I'm Just Too Tired To Cook!

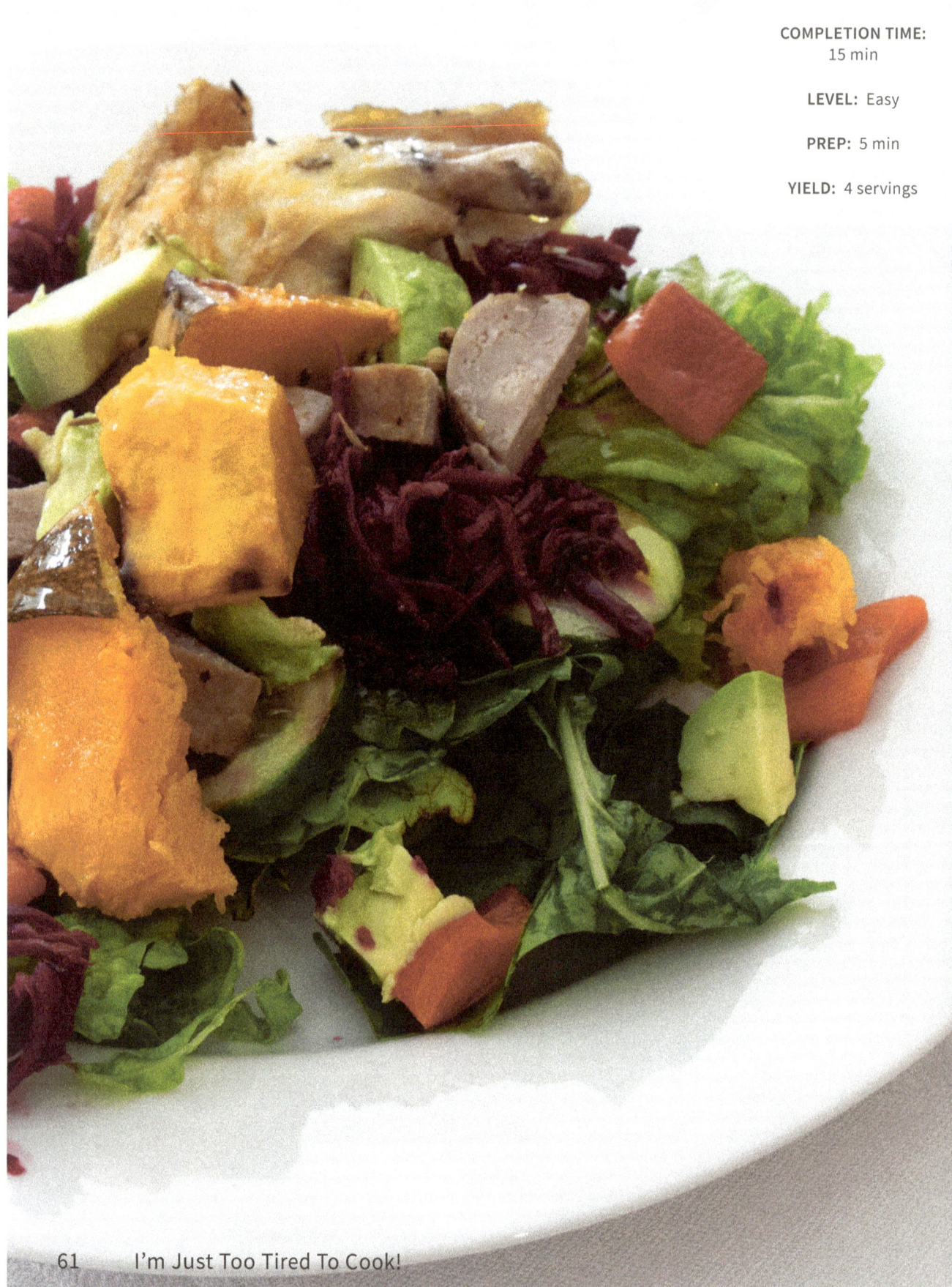

COMPLETION TIME: 15 min

LEVEL: Easy

PREP: 5 min

YIELD: 4 servings

Suddenly salad

Gluten Free Nut Free Dairy Free Sugar Free

Salads are commonly eaten before or with the main meal.
This enables the acidic dressing and enzyme-rich raw and fermented foods to support digestion of the main course which follows.
Microbe-rich fermented foods eaten with protein will help to maintain a balanced microbiota.

Ingredients

fresh seasonal lettuce greens
chopped parsley
fresh basil
avocado
fresh or semi dried tomatoes
bottled olives drained
bottles capers drained
Fermented veg (p24)
olive oil
lemons quartered
left over roast meat or poultry and roast vegetables
salt and pepper to taste.

Method

1. Toss it all together and enjoy

Fermented veg
Page 24

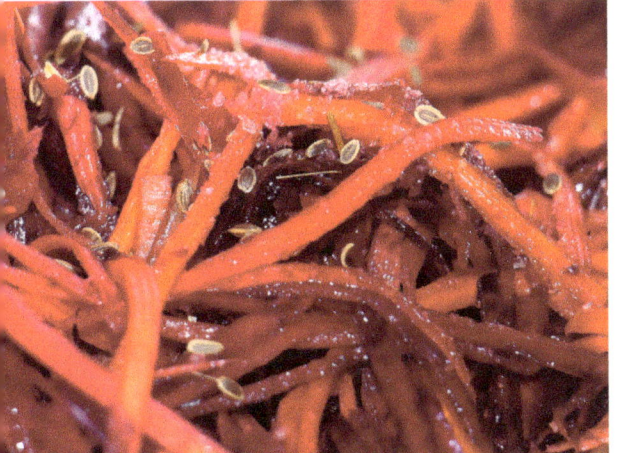

Right now roast
Page 63

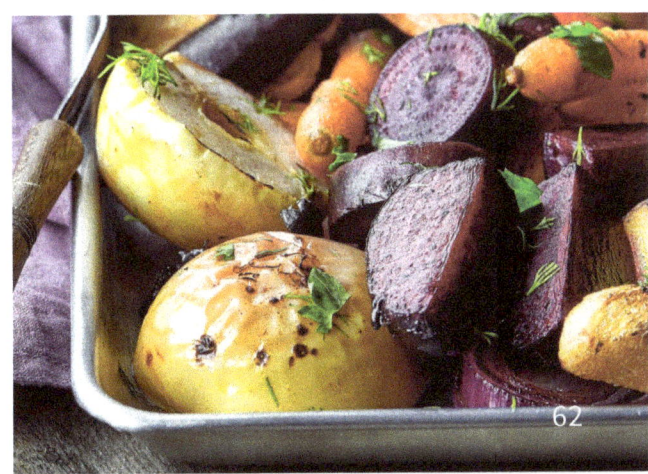

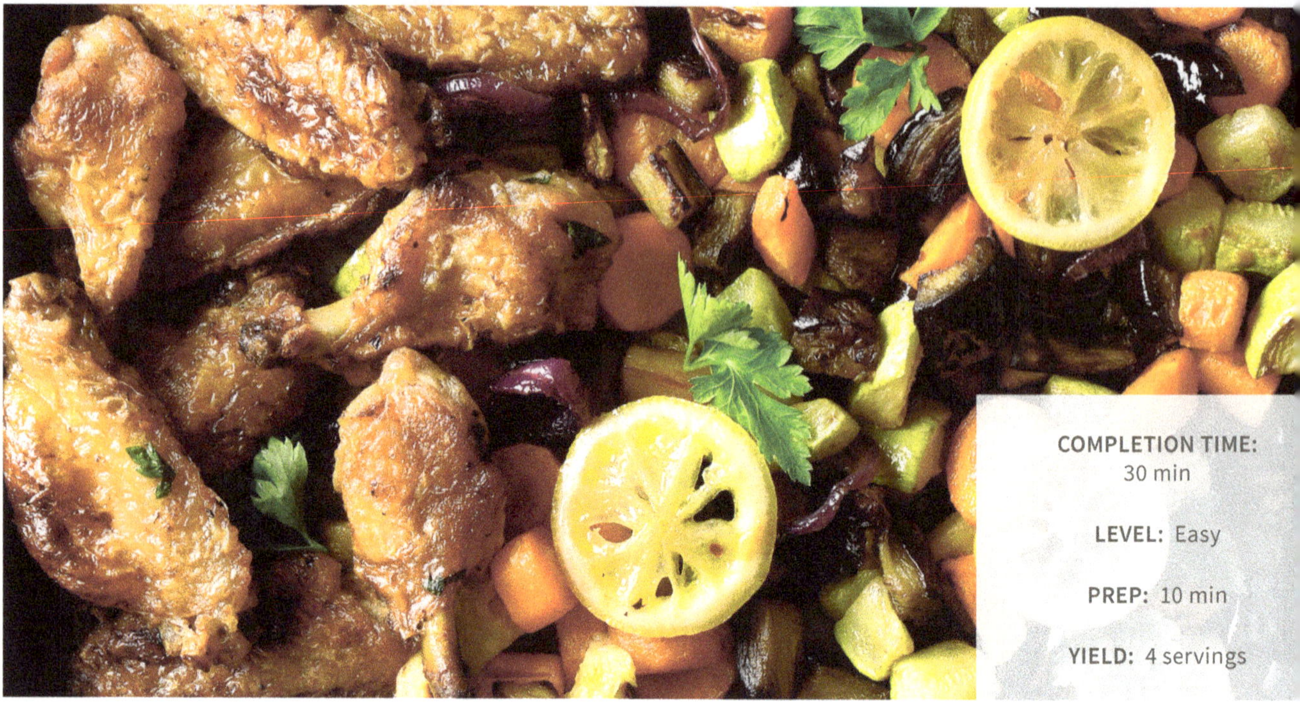

COMPLETION TIME: 30 min

LEVEL: Easy

PREP: 10 min

YIELD: 4 servings

Right now roast

Gluten Free   Nut Free   Dairy Free   Sugar Free

Prepare a large tray and keep on hand for Suddenly salad (p62), Pizza (p54), Not fast enough five minute casserole (p60), Resuscitating Thai curry (p64) or Moussaka (p48).

Ingredients

roughly chopped low thiol vegetables including;
baby beets
carrots
pumpkin
parsnip
potato

chicken nibblets, wings or drums

organic olive oil and ghee

dried thyme

salt and peppe

Method

1. Heat the oil and ghee in a large baking tray in a hot fan forced oven
2. Carefully transfer the meat and vegetables onto the tray with the salt, pepper and herbs
3. Mix around to coat
4. Roast for around 25 minutes or until golden brown

Resuscitating Thai curry

Ingredients

Low thiol Thai curry paste (p20)
olive oil
coconut milk
left over roast vegetables
left over roast meat or fresh fillets of fish

Method

1. Heat the olive oil and warm the paste until fragrant
2. Add the remaining ingredients and warm through
3. Serve with boiled rice

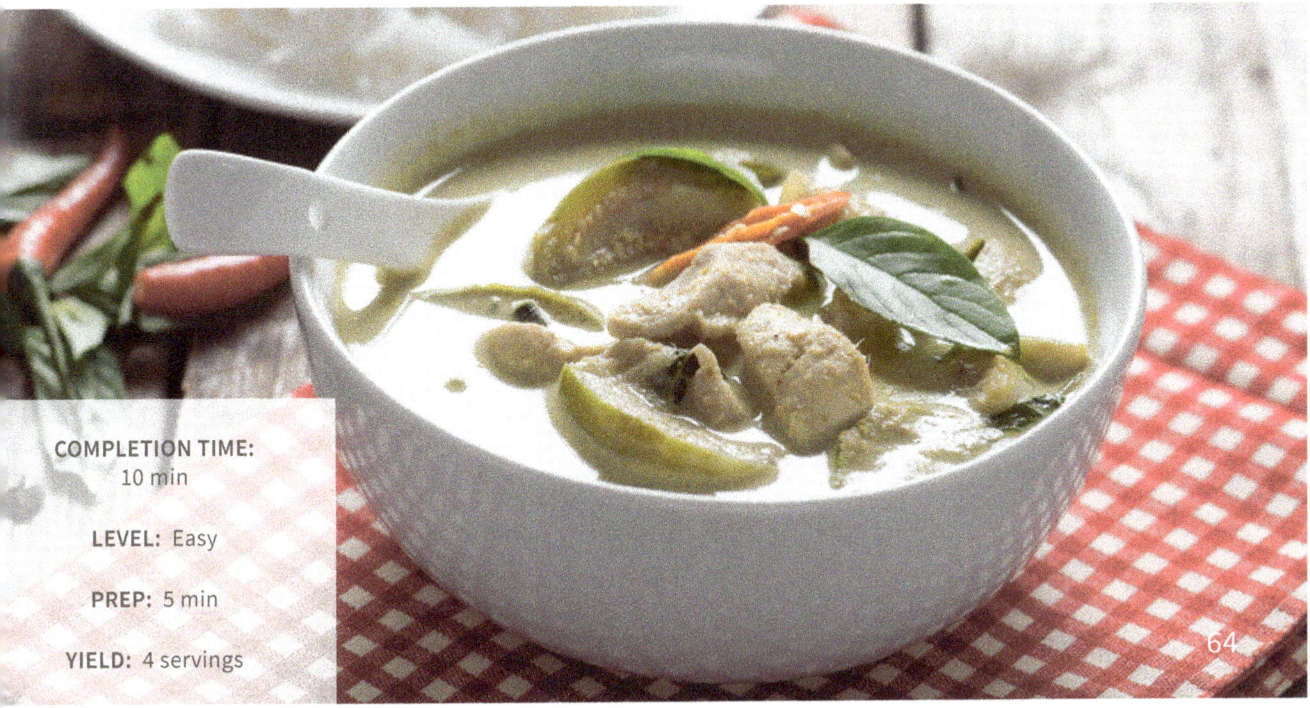

COMPLETION TIME: 10 min

LEVEL: Easy

PREP: 5 min

YIELD: 4 servings

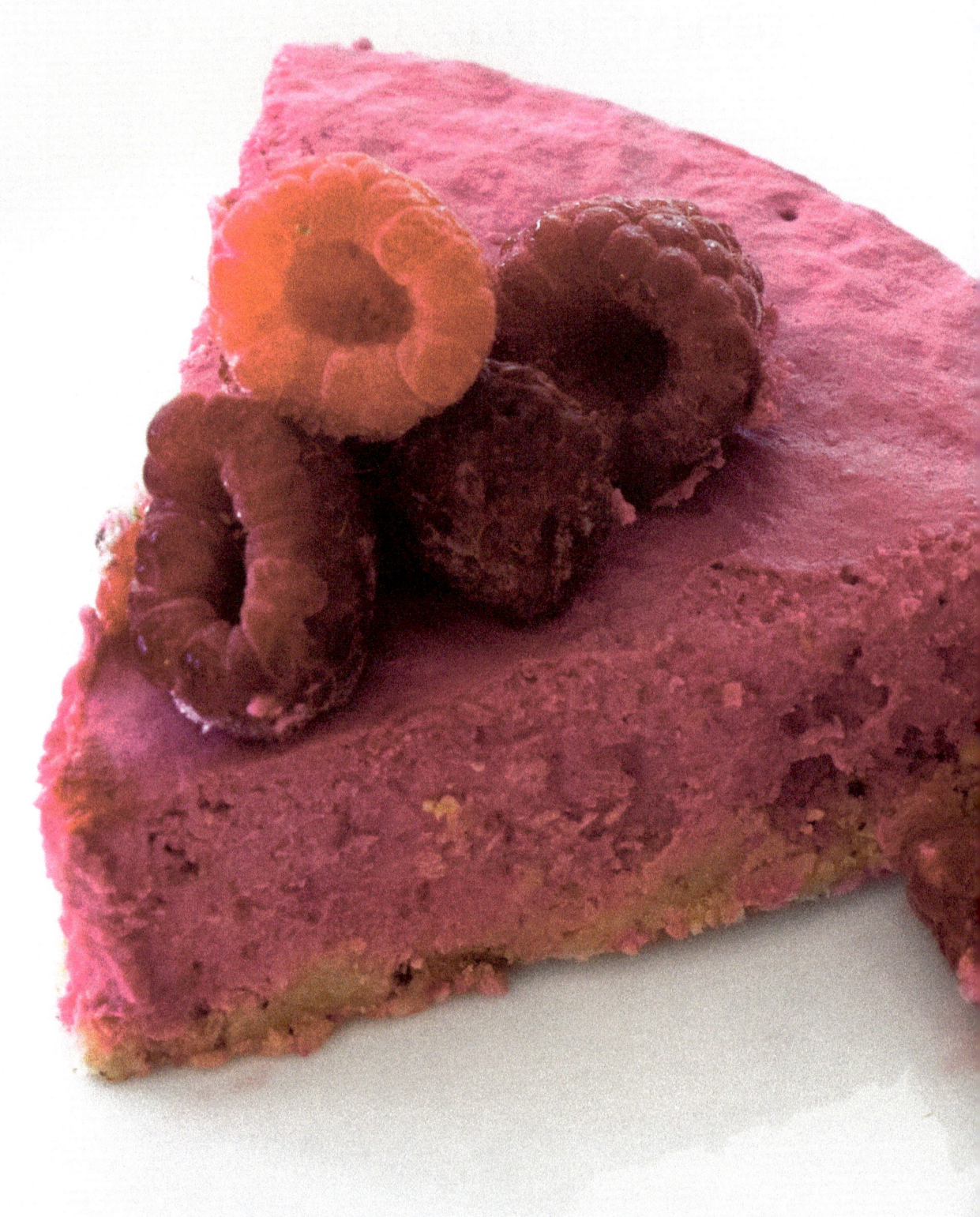

Raw raspberry & beetroot no-cheese cake p69

You're Sweet Enough

to tempt your guests and delight your taste buds

Cashew custard	68	Raw raspberry & beetroot no-cheese cake	69
Whipped creamy coconut	68	Apple crumble	71
Jillaine's raw honey drizzle	68	Lemon spice gummies	72

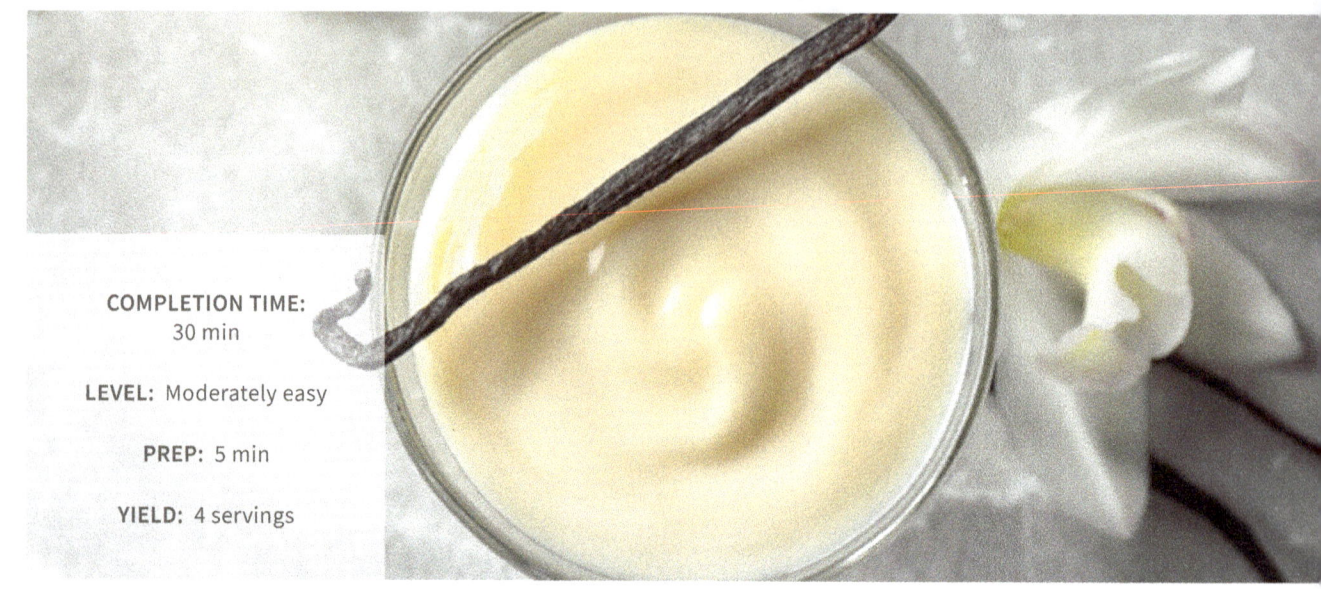

COMPLETION TIME: 30 min

LEVEL: Moderately easy

PREP: 5 min

YIELD: 4 servings

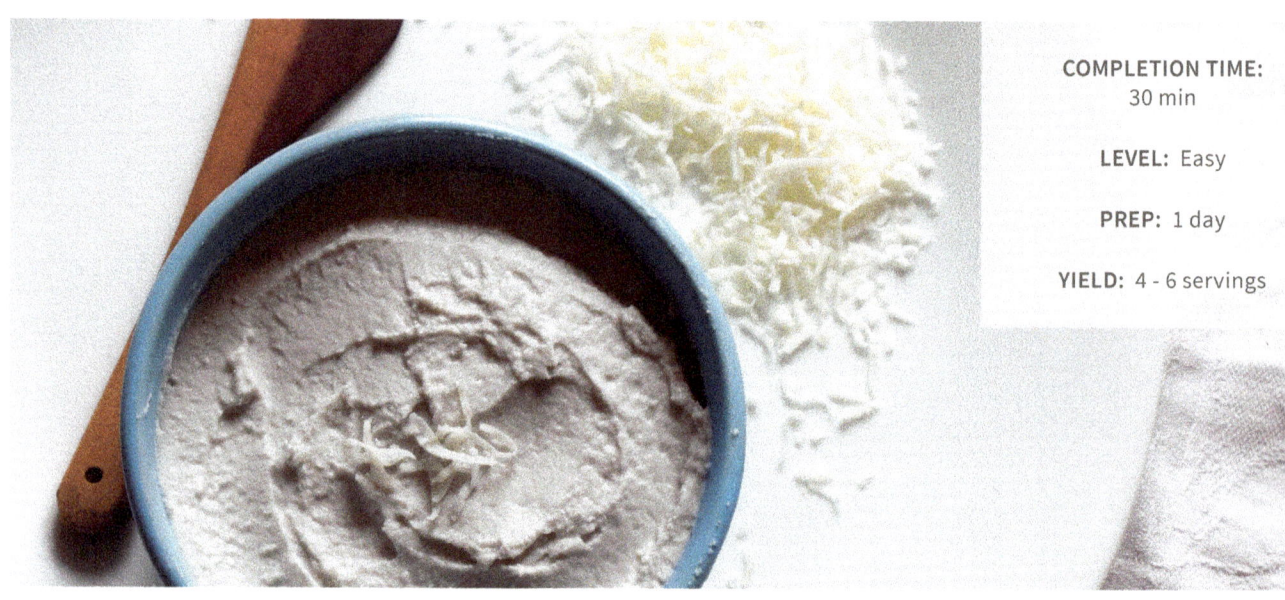

COMPLETION TIME: 30 min

LEVEL: Easy

PREP: 1 day

YIELD: 4 - 6 servings

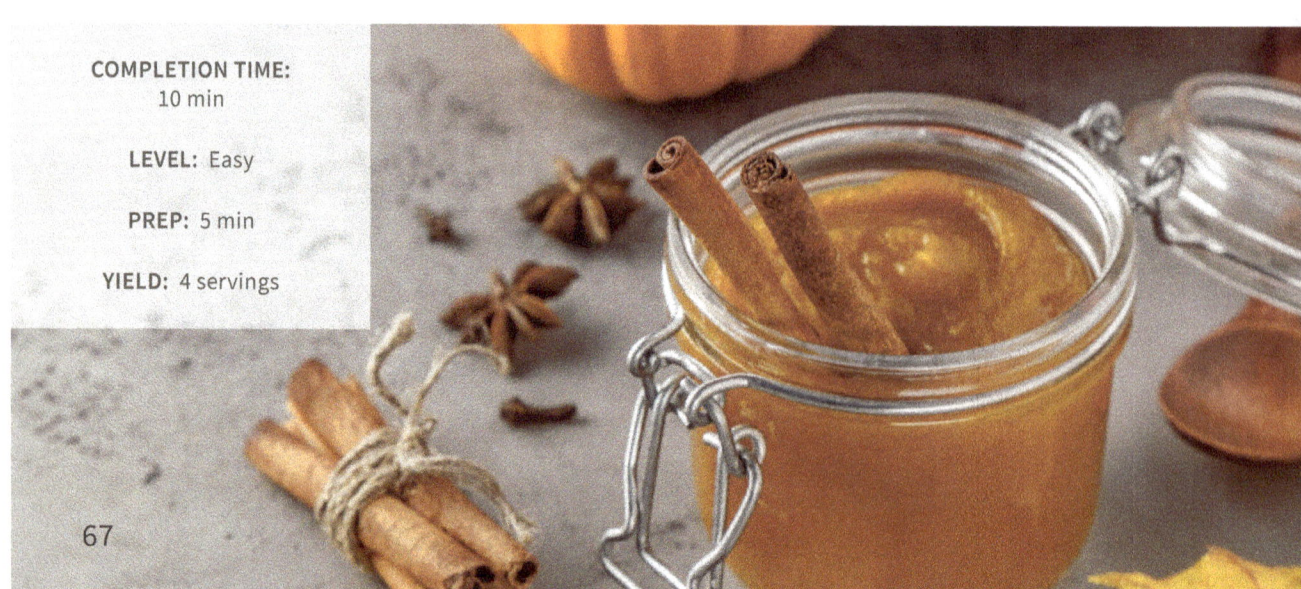

COMPLETION TIME: 10 min

LEVEL: Easy

PREP: 5 min

YIELD: 4 servings

Cashew custard

Ingredients

1 cup activated* cashew *Nut milk (p95)*

1 1/2 tsp tapioca starch

2 tsp maple syrup

1 tsp vanilla essence

a pinch of salt

Method

1. Place the milk into a small saucepan over a low to moderate heat
2. Whisk in the tapioca starch and add the salt, vanilla and sweetener
3. Continue whisking over a moderate heat until the mixture begins to thicken slightly
4. Remove from the heat and continue to whisk
5. Serve immediately or store in an air tight container in the fridge for up to 3 days

For more information about why it is important to activate nuts, see page xxiv

Whipped creamy coconut

Ingredients

1 tin full-fat coconut milk refrigerated overnight

1 tsp vanilla extract

1 Tbs maple syrup or raw honey

Method

1. Place mixing bowl into the freezer to chill 10 minutes before use
2. Turn the can upside down and open the bottom. Pour off the liquid portion (use in a smoothie)
3. Empty the remaining solids from the tin into the chilled mixing bowl
4. Use a hand beater or electric mixer to whip the coconut cream until it becomes light and fluffy
5. Mix in the sweetener and vanilla
6. Serve immediately or store in an air tight container in the fridge for up to 3 days

Jillaine's raw honey drizzle

Ingredients

1/2 cup honey - preferably local and raw/unpasteurised

1/2 cup ghee

Pinch of salt

1/2 tsp *Sweet spice blend (p100)* (optional)

Method

1. In a small saucepan warm the above ingredients gently over a low heat until the honey is soft and the ghee is melted
2. Remove from the heat and whisk in a chilled bowl to combine
3. Store in the fridge. Warm and whisk before use
4. Pour over *Seed loaf (p84)*, *Creamy spiced porridge (p11)* or *Muffins (p75)*

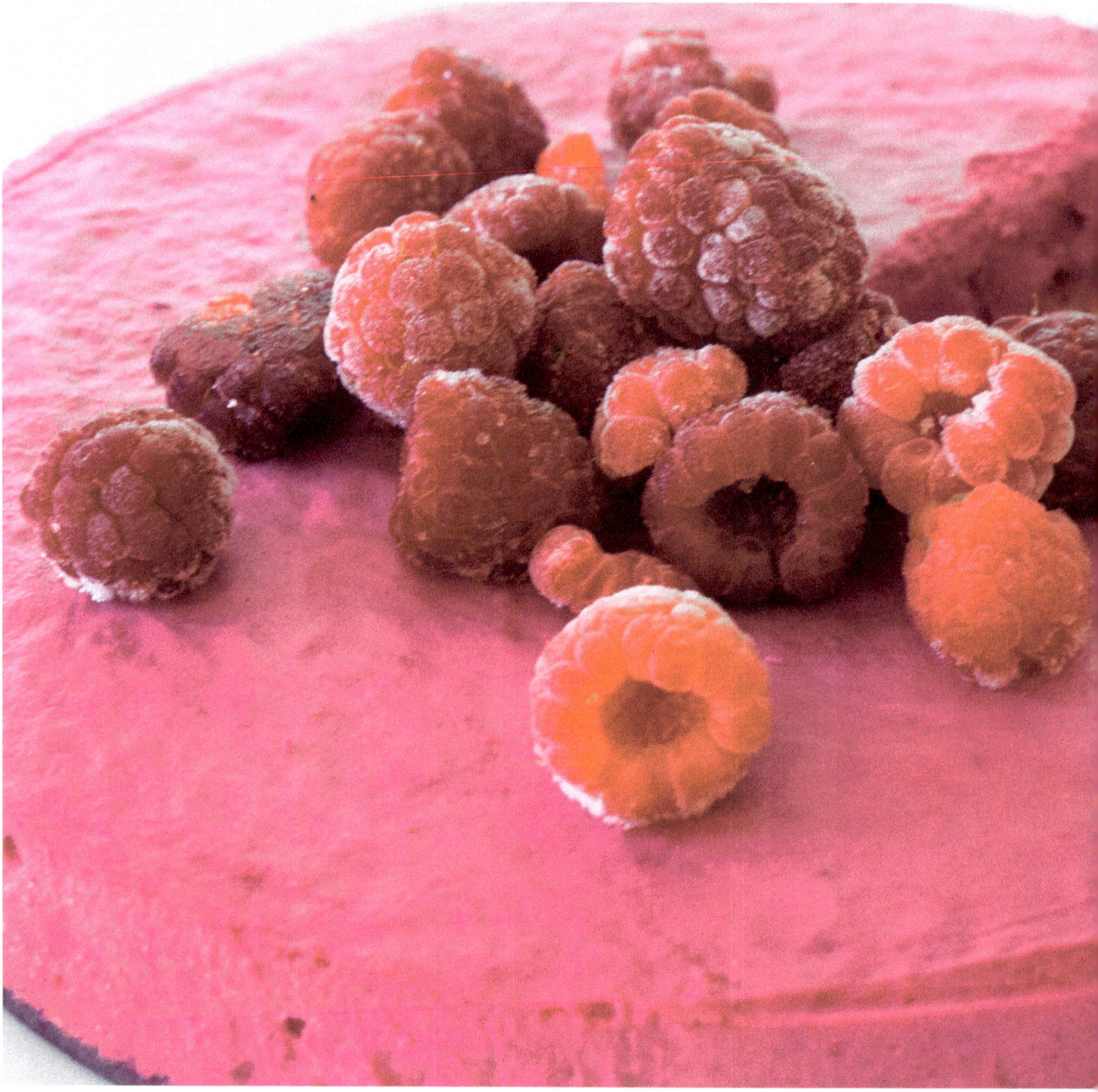

Raw raspberry & beetroot no-cheese cake

Gluten Free   Vegetarian   Dairy Free   Sugar Free

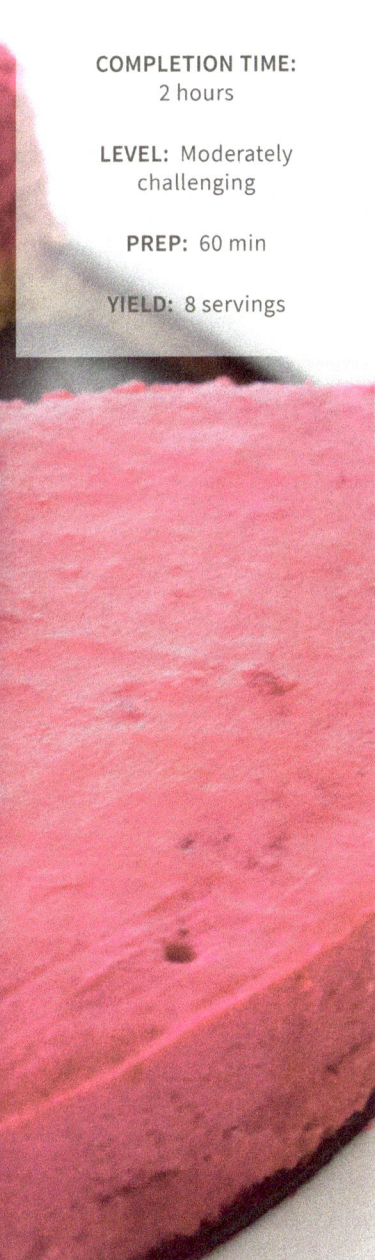

COMPLETION TIME:
2 hours

LEVEL: Moderately challenging

PREP: 60 min

YIELD: 8 servings

Base

Ingredients

1/2 cup raw soaked (cover with boiled water for an hour) and drained cashews or almonds or pecans*

1 medjool date pitted

1 Tbs maple syrup

1 Tbs coconut oil melted

2 tsp *Sweet spice blend* *(p100)*

Method

1. Blend the base ingredients together in a food process
2. Transfer to a large spring form pan which has been greased using melted coconut oil
3. Wet your hands and press the base out evenly over the pan
4. Place in the freezer whilst preparing the filling

Filling

Ingredients

1 cup raw, soaked (cover with boiled water for an hour) and drained cashews*

1/3 cup freshly squeezed lemon juice (2 large lemons)

1 medium raw beet, peeled and roughly chopped

1 cup fresh or thawed frozen raspberries

1/4 cup coconut oil melted

1/2 cup coconut yogurt

1/2 cup coconut cream (full fat 100%)

1/4 cup pure maple syrup

Method

1. Place the drained cashews in a blender together with the lemon juice, melted coconut oil, raspberries, raw beet, yogurt ,coconut cream and maple syrup
2. Blend together until very smooth
3. Pour the filling over the base and return the tin to the freezer for 1 - 2 hours or until set
4. To serve: allow the no-cheese cake to soften at room temperature for
   15 - 20 minutes
5. Serve with *Whipped creamy coconut* *(p68)*

*For more information about why it is important to activate nuts, see page xxiv

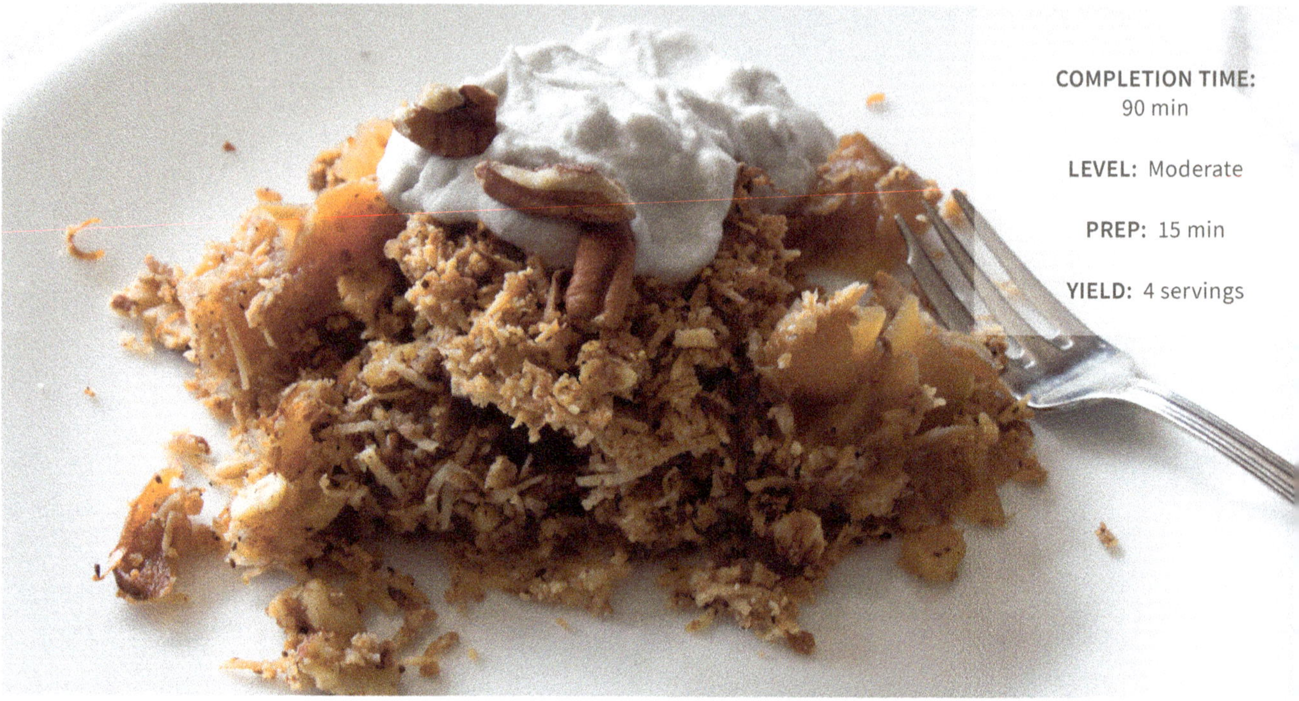

COMPLETION TIME: 90 min

LEVEL: Moderate

PREP: 15 min

YIELD: 4 servings

Apple crumble

Gluten Free | Vegetarian | Dairy Free | Sugar Free

Ingredients

Apple Base:
6 fresh fresh sweet apples
1 tsp *Sweet spice blend (p100)*

Crumble Topping:
1/3 cup melted ghee
1/3 cup almond meal
1 cup activated* almonds chopped
1 Tbs Sweet Spice Blend
1 tsp 100% vanilla extract
1 cup of desiccated or shredded coconut
1 Tbs rapadura sugar OR 1/2 a dropper full of vanilla stevia liquid (sugar-free option)
pinch of Himalayan salt

Method

1. Preheat oven to 180°C or 350°F.
2. Grease a medium sized casserole dish or pyrex pie dish with ghee
3. Peel, core and dice the apples then place them into the dish
4. Sprinkle mixed spice over apples and mix well
5. Combine the remaining dry ingredients in a large bowl
6. Mix the vanilla and stevia liquid into the melted ghee and mix through the dry ingredients
7. Sprinkle the crumble over apples then bake in the preheated oven for 15 minutes
8. Remove the dish from the oven. Cover with baking paper and a layer of foil
9. Return to the oven for a further 40 minutes or until apples are cooked and crumble browned
10. Serve warm with coconut yogurt or *Cashew custard (p68)*, or *Whipped creamy coconut (p68)*

Variation: Add 1/2 cup blueberries or 1/2 cup stewed drained apricots or a handful of soaked raisins.

*For more information about why it is important to activate nuts, see page xxiv

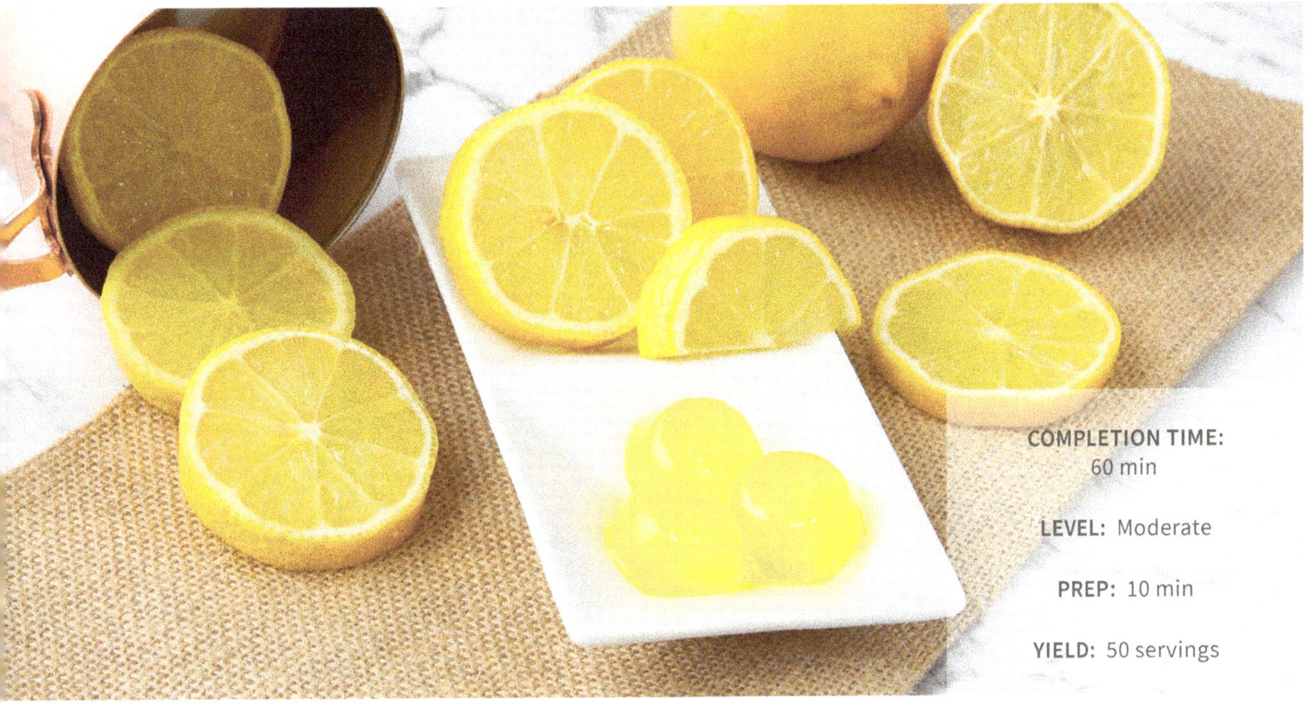

COMPLETION TIME: 60 min

LEVEL: Moderate

PREP: 10 min

YIELD: 50 servings

Lemon spice gummies

Gluten Free   Nut Free   Vegetarian   Dairy Free   Sugar Free

The essential oils in this recipe have anti fungal, antibacterial and anti-inflammatory functions. I like to recommend this recipe to parents who are looking to supplement their children with essential nutrients commonly depleted by heavy metal toxicity. Zinc, Vitamin C, Magnesium and vitamin E can be mixed into the recipe once the liquid has been strained. Speak to your health care practitioner to ensure the correct dosage for your child.

Ingredients

400ml filtered water

5 cm piece ginger finely grated

1/2 cinnamon stick

3 whole cloves

50g powdered grass fed gelatin

3 tbsp lemon juice

3 tbsp manuka honey

2 drops lemongrass essential oil

1 drop clove essential oil

2 drops lemon essential oil

NOTE: Makes 50 gummies
Recipe Author: Danielle O'Donoghue

Method

1. Place 200 ml of filtered water, chopped ginger, cinnamon stick and clove into a small saucepan and bring to a rapid boil with the lid on. Reduce the heat and simmer for 10 mins
2. Turn off the heat and allow to stand with the lid on for 45mins
3. Meanwhile sprinkle the gelatine powder over the remaining 200ml of water, stir well and allow to stand for at least 5 mins. This allows the gelatine granules to expand and soften
4. Heat the spiced water back to a gentle simmer over low heat. Stir in the gelatine mixture and continue stirring for about 3 mins. Once the gelatine has completely dissolved remove from heat and add the honey, lemon juice and essential oils. Stir well to dissolve the honey completely
5. Pour the liquid through a strainer to remove the spices
6. Fill silicone moulds with the mixture and place into the fridge or freezer to set. Once set remove the gummies and store in an airtight container. They should last up to 2 weeks

You're Sweet Enough

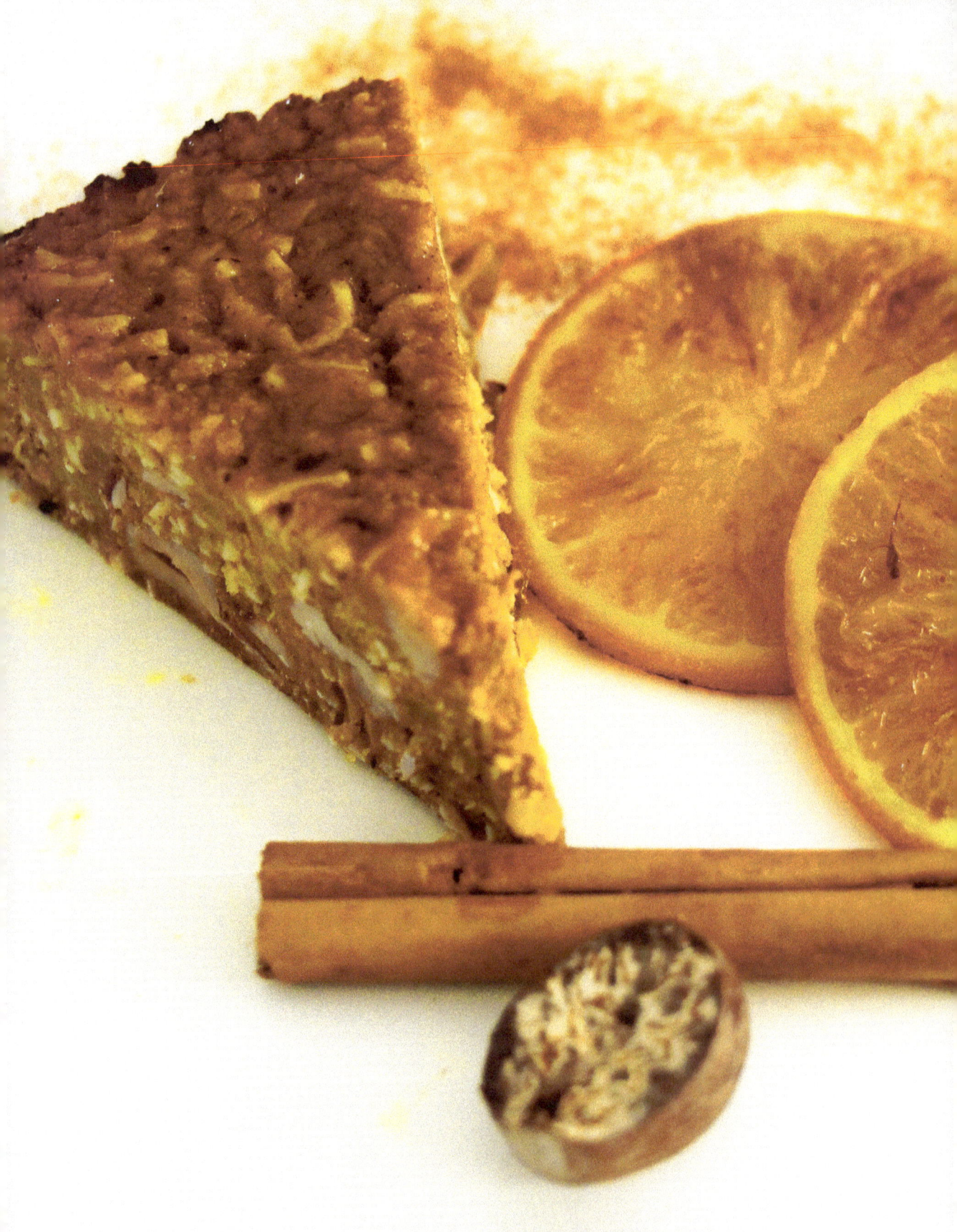

Muffins	75
Low thiol & gluten-free flour	75
Anzac cookies	77
Gluten-free banana bread	78
Pumpkin & ginger tart	79
Ginger snaps	81
Spicy pumpkin cake	82
Seed loaf olive & rosemary or fig & sweet spice	84
Spicy seed crackers	85
Herbed seed crackers	85
Cumin flatbread	87
Chilli lime sweet potato chips	88

The Way To My Heart
gluten-free baking

Muffins

Ingredients

3 cups pre-soaked and dried* rolled oats

3/4 cup raw activated* cashews

1 cup of grated or drained stewed apples

2 Tbs honey or maple syrup

1 tsp vanilla extract

1 tsp *Sweet spice blend (p100)*

1 1/2 tsp baking soda

1 1/4 cups water

1/4 cup coconut yogurt

1/2 cup *Kombucha (p93)*

Method

1. Place all ingredients into a food processor or blender and blend until the cashews are smooth. Transfer to a covered bowl and allow to sit for around 4 hours
2. Preheat oven to 180°C or 350°F
3. Place batter into paper-lined muffin tins and bake for about 20 minutes or until a skewer comes out clean

Variation: 1 cup fresh blueberries, or 1 cup fresh raspberries or 1 cup of soaked and drained chopped dates.

*For more information about why it is important to soak oats and activate nuts, see page xxiv

Low thiol & gluten-free flour

Ingredients

1 1/2 cups sorghum flour

1 1/2 cups teff flour

1 cup tapioca flour/ starch

1 cup green banana flour

1 1/2 tsp xanthan gum

Method

1. Mix all of the ingredients together and store in an airtight container

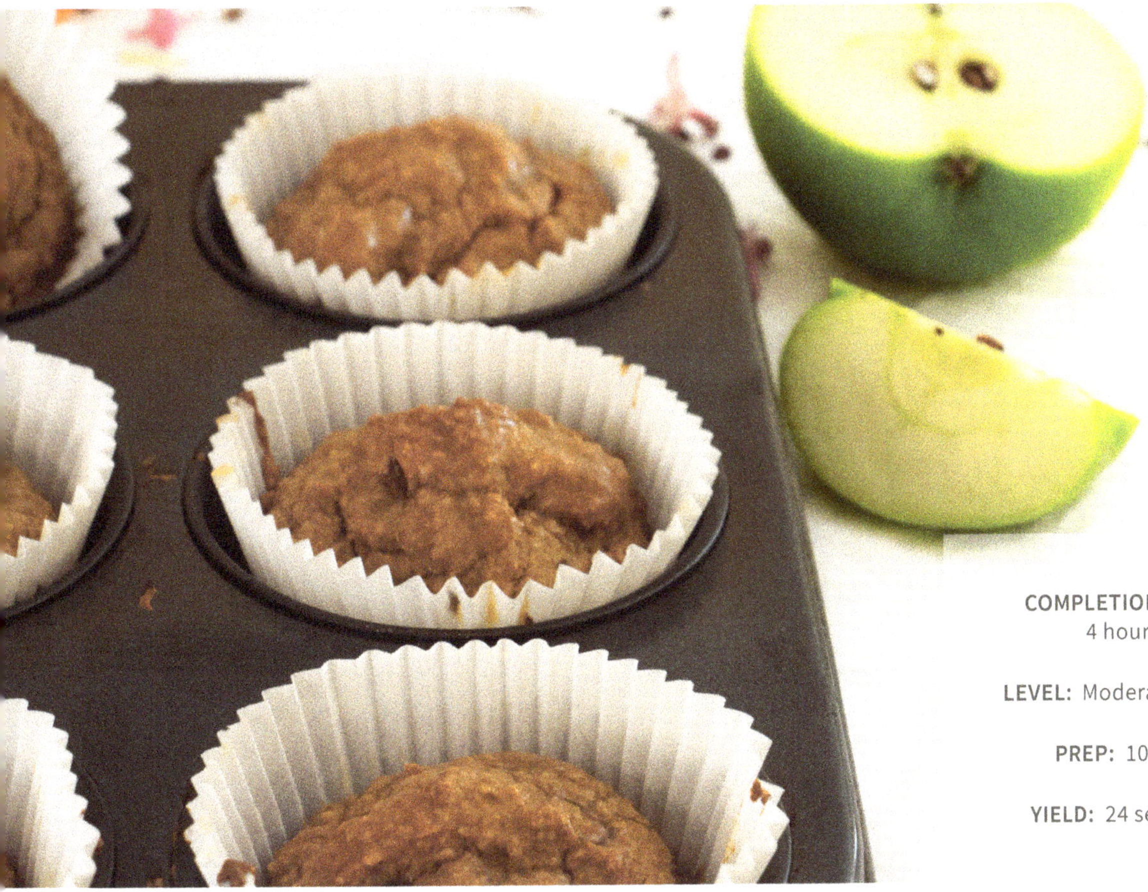

COMPLETION TIME:
4 hours

LEVEL: Moderately easy

PREP: 10 min

YIELD: 24 servings

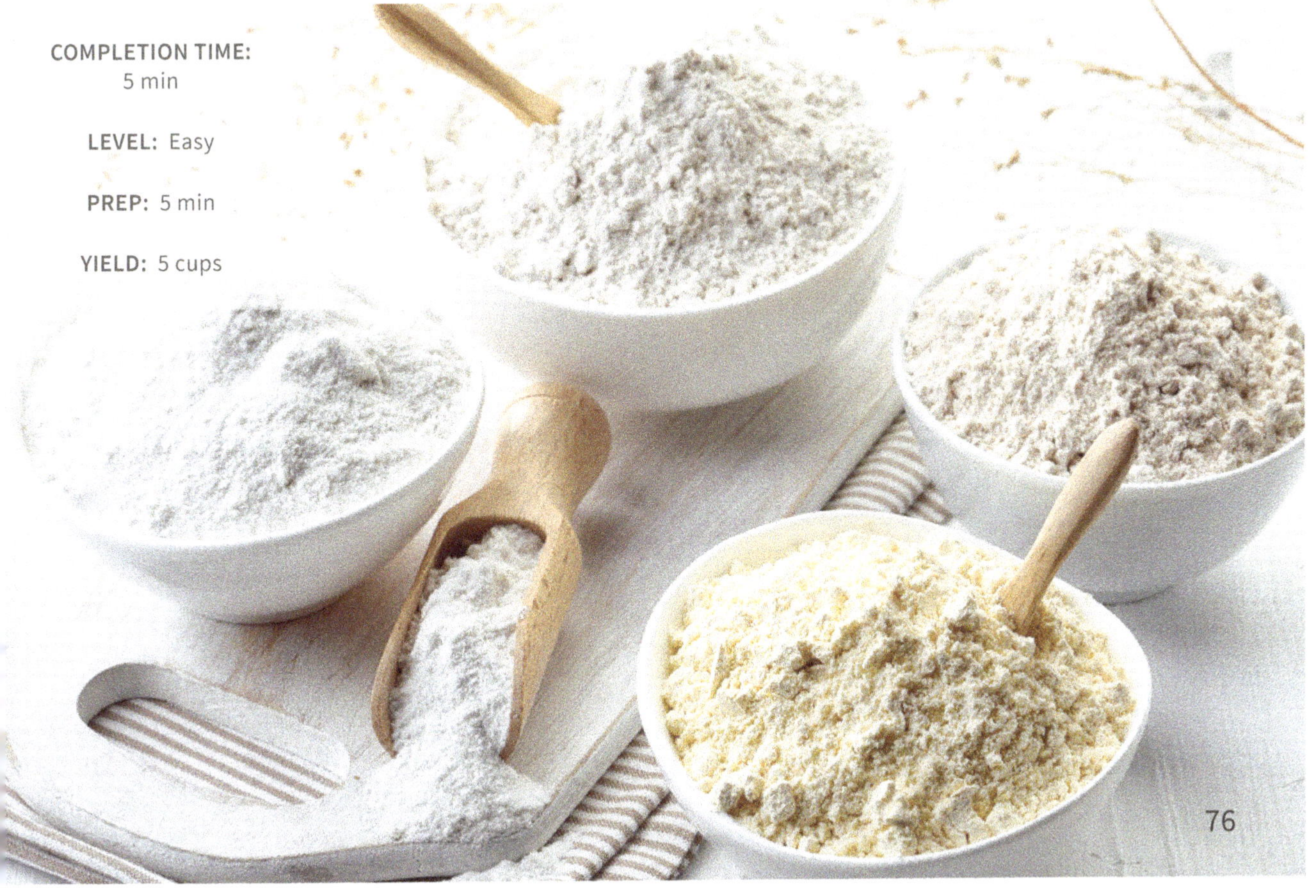

COMPLETION TIME:
5 min

LEVEL: Easy

PREP: 5 min

YIELD: 5 cups

COMPLETION TIME:
45 min

LEVEL: Moderately easy

PREP: 1 day

YIELD: 14 servings

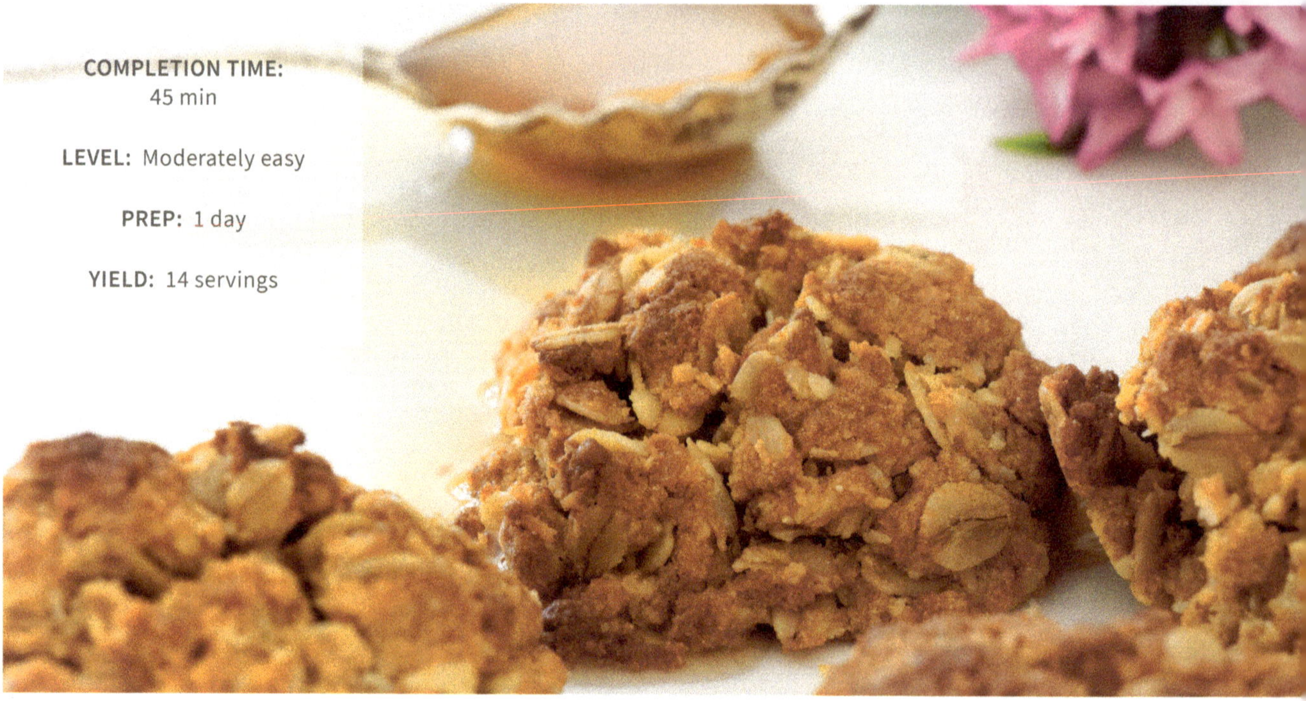

Anzac cookies

 Gluten Free   Nut Free   Vegetarian   Dairy Free

Grains contain phytic acid which blocks the absorption of important minerals needed to displace heavy metals and therefore reduce ongoing uptake. To overcome this issue soak the rolled oats and sorghum flour in warm pure filtered water and dry.

Ingredients

1 cup pre-soaked and dried* rolled oats

1 cup pre-soaked and dried* sorghum flour

1 Tbs rapadura or coconut sugar

1 cup shredded coconut

1/2 tsp xanthan gum

125g melted ghee

1 Tbs honey

1 Tbs boiling water

1/2 tsp aluminium free baking soda

Method

1. Preheat oven to 160°C or 320°F.
2. Place the oats, flour, sugar, coconut and xanthan gum in a bowl and stir to combine
3. Place the ghee and honey in a small saucepan over low heat and stir until butter is melted.
4. Place the water and baking soda in a bowl and stir to combine. Add to the butter mixture and combine
5. Pour the butter mixture over the flour mixture and stir well to combine
6. Place a Tbs of the mixture on to baking trays lined with baking paper, allowing room for spread.
7. Flatten slightly and bake for 10-12 mins or until golden

*For each cup of oats/flour, use 1/2 cup of pure filtered water and 1 Tbs of lemon juice or kombucha.
In a large bowl, stir together the oats/flour and water mixture, cover with a cloth and allow to sit in a warm place for 12 – 24 hours. This will break down the phytic acid.
Spread the soaked grain mixture onto dehydrator trays and dry the mixture on the warmest setting until completely dry. Around 12 hours. I recommend Excalibur or similar dehydrator to ensure that the grain is crispy, crumbly dry for storage purposes. You can use your dehydrator to dry soaked nuts and seeds and your surplus produce.
*For more information about why it is important to soak grains, see page xxiv

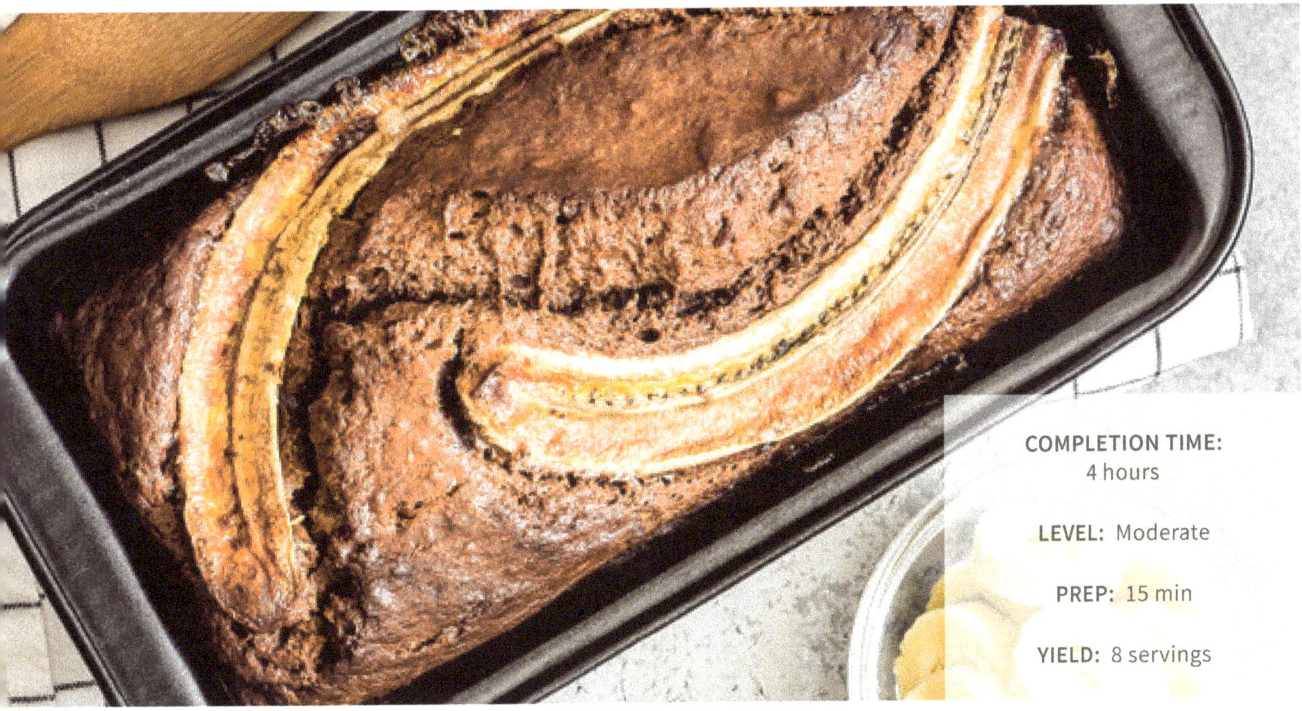

COMPLETION TIME: 4 hours

LEVEL: Moderate

PREP: 15 min

YIELD: 8 servings

Gluten-free banana bread

 Gluten Free Nut Free Vegetarian Dairy Free

Ingredients

1 3/4 cup low thiol & gluten-free flour *(p75)*

1 tsp aluminium-free baking soda

1/2 tsp baking powder

1/2 tsp himalayan salt

1/4 cup rapadura or coconut sugar

1/3 cup melted coconut oil

2 ripe bananas peeled

1 tsp vanilla extract

1 tsp apple cider vinegar

1/4 cup pure water

2 tsp *Sweet spice blend (p100)*

Method

1. Preheat oven to 175°C or 350°F
2. Line a loaf tin with greased baking paper
3. In a food processor blend the bananas and coconut oil together
4. Blend in the sugar, vanilla, water and vinegar
5. In a separate bowl sift together the flour, salt, baking soda and baking powder
6. Mix the wet ingredients into the dry ingredients, stir to combine
7. Cover the batter with a cloth and allow to sit in a warm place for 2-4 hours
8. Pour the batter into the baking tin and bake for 40 - 45 minutes or until a toothpick inserted into the middle of the loaf comes out clean
9. Allow to cool in the pan for 30 minutes then lift the loaf out onto a rack to cool before slicing

Pumpkin & ginger tart

Ingredients

Short Crust Pastry

2 cups *Low thiol & gluten-free flour (p75)*

1 tsp aluminium-free baking soda

1/4 cup coconut sugar

1/2 tsp xanthan gum

1/4 tsp salt

140g cold ghee

1/4 cup dry baked pumpkin puree

1 tsp melted ghee or butter to grease the pan

Filling

2 cups roasted pumpkin, cooled and pureed

1/4 cup coconut sugar

2 tsp aluminium-free baking powder

1 Tbs water

1 1/2 cups coconut cream

6 Tbs activated* almond or cashew cream

2 Tbs *Low thiol & gluten-free flour (p75)*

2 tsp *Sweet spice blend (p100)*

2 tsp finely grated ginger

Method

Pastry

1. Place the flour, baking soda, coconut sugar, xanthan gum and salt into food processor or bowl
2. Pulse to combine
3. Add the cold ghee and process for a few minutes to resemble bread crumbs
4. Add the cooked pumpkin and mix briefly until just combined
5. Turn the dough out onto a clean surface and work the dough together with your hands to form a smooth ball
6. Wrap in cling wrap and place in the fridge for 15 minutes

Filling

7. Place the pumpkin, coconut sugar, coconut cream, cashew cream, flour, spices and ginger into a food processor and process until just combined

Assemble

8. Preheat oven to 200°C or 400°F
9. Prepare a 24 cm fluted pie dish or removable base tart tin by brushing thoroughly with melted butter or ghee
10. Roll out the pastry between two sheets of lightly floured baking paper until 3mm or 1/8 inch thick
11. Invert into the pie dish or removable base tart tin and trim. If the pastry is breaking you may find it easier to wet your hands and work the pastry into the tin by hand
12. Prick the base and sides of the pastry, line with non-stick baking paper and fill with baking weights or rice
13. Bake the pastry case for 10 minutes, remove the weights and paper add the filling
14. Reduce oven temperature to 170°C or 340°F and bake for 25 - 30 minutes or until the filling is just set
15. Serve with *Whipped creamy coconut (p68)*

*For more information about why it is important to activate nuts, see page xxiv

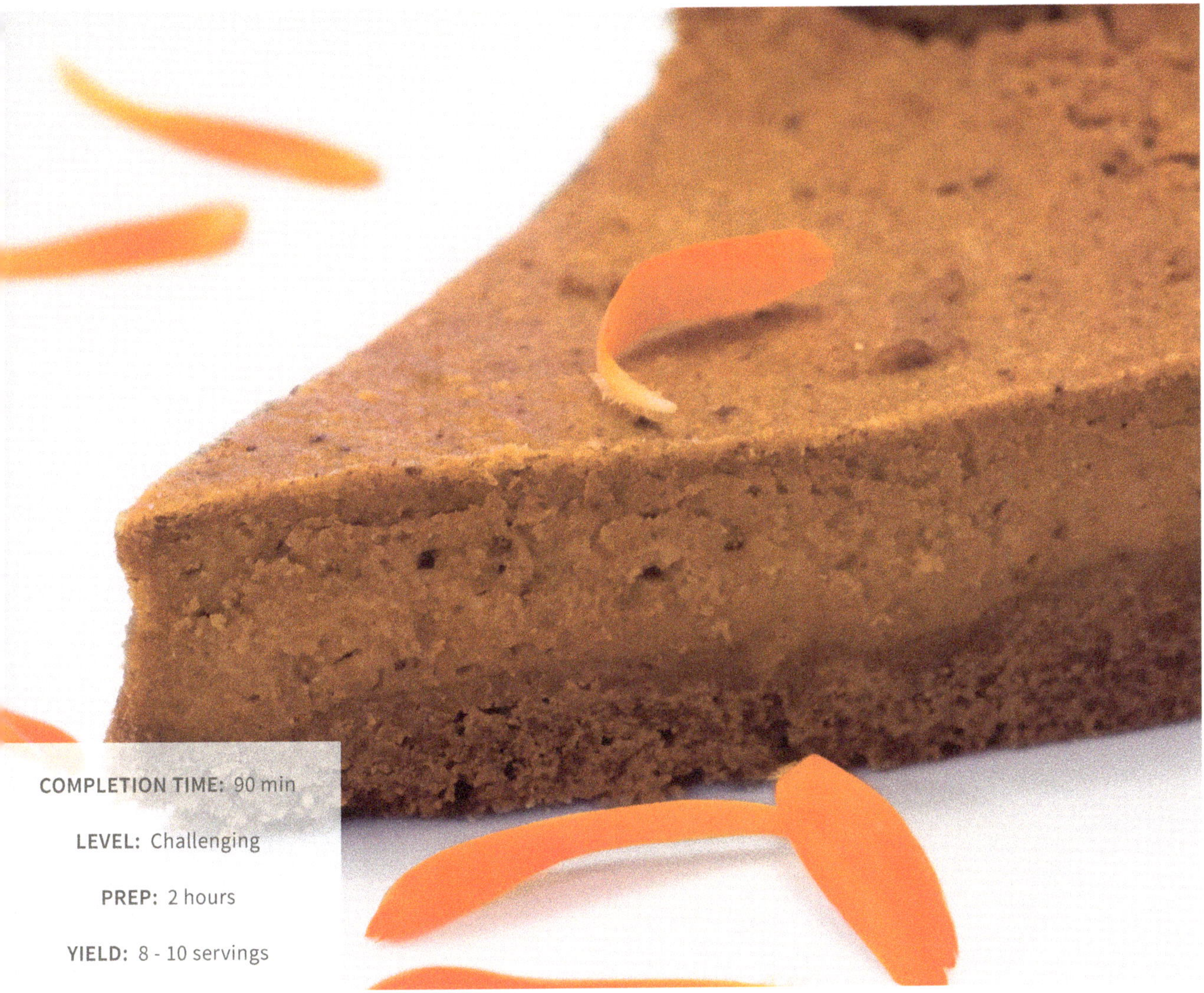

COMPLETION TIME: 90 min

LEVEL: Challenging

PREP: 2 hours

YIELD: 8 - 10 servings

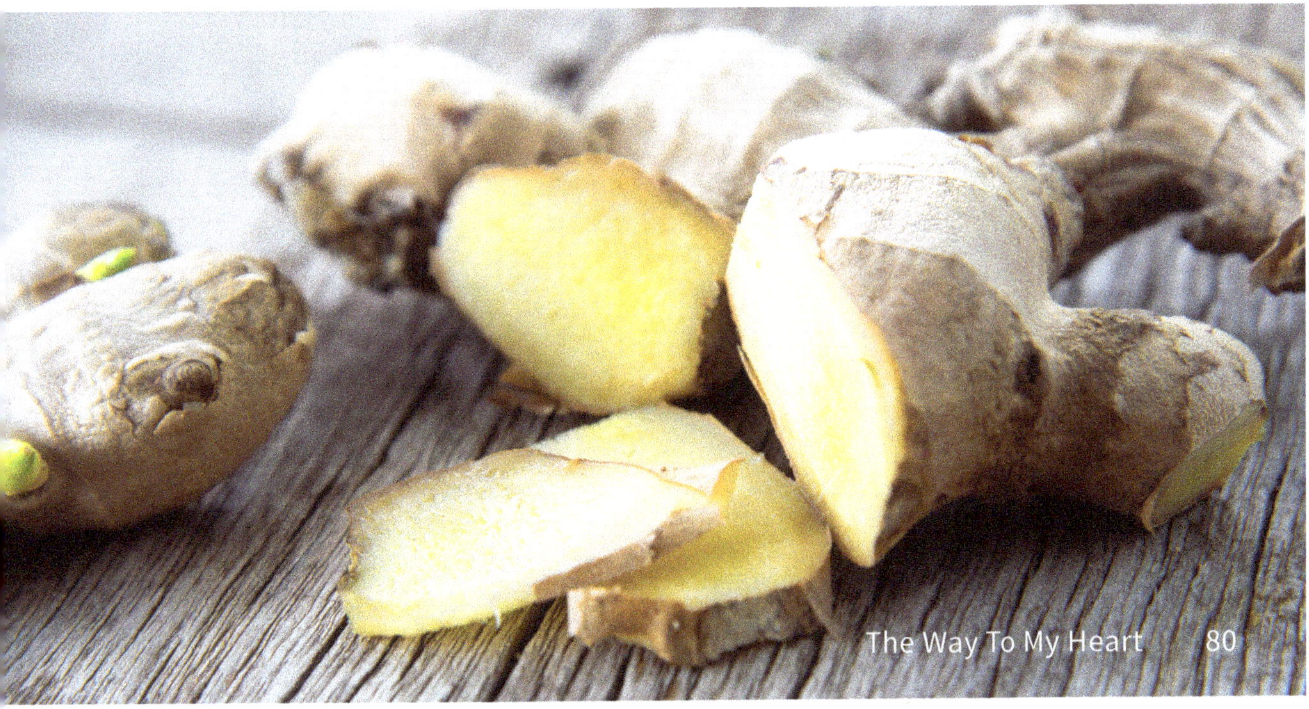

COMPLETION TIME: 4 hours

LEVEL: Moderate

PREP: 10 min

YIELD: 24 servings

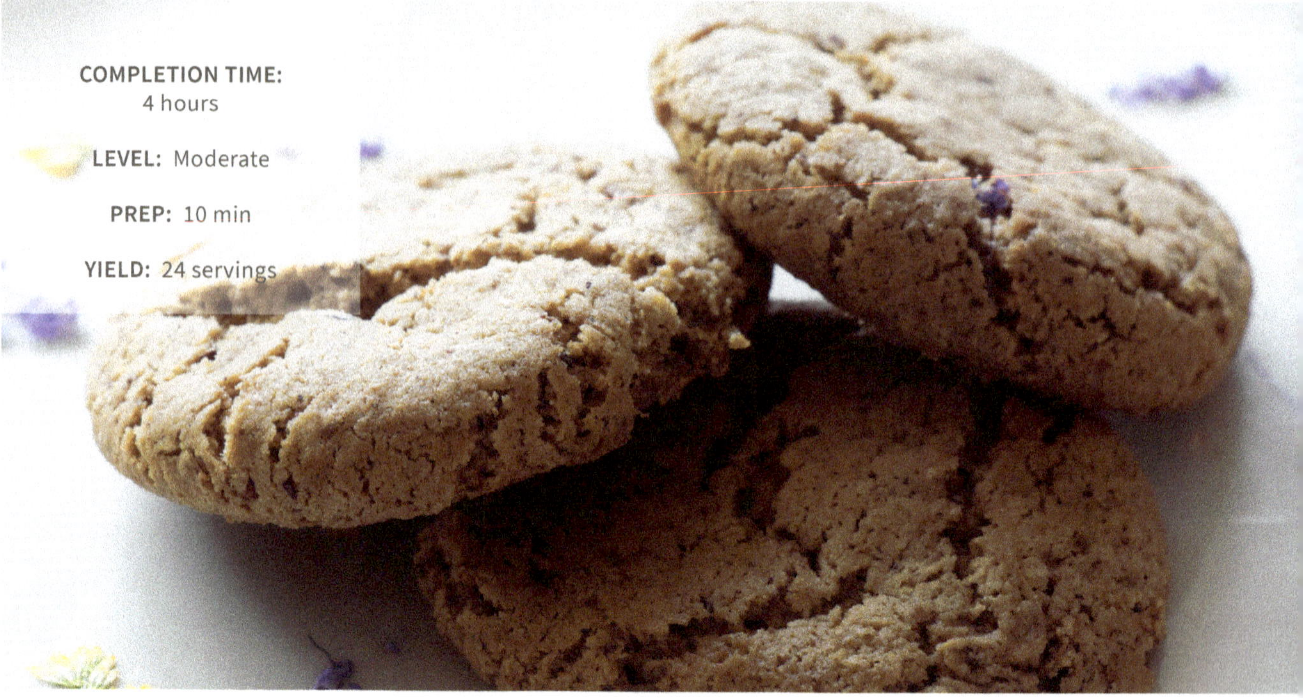

Ginger snaps

 Gluten Free   Nut Free   Vegetarian   Dairy Free

Ingredients

60g ghee

1/4 cup maple syrup or honey

2 tsp *Sweet spice blend (p100)*

pinch Himalayan salt

1 tsp aluminium-free baking soda

1 1/4 cups *Low thiol & gluten-free flour (p75)*

1 Tbs finely grated fresh ginger

1/4 cup rapadura sugar or coconut sugar

Method

1. Preheat oven to 160°C or 320°F
2. Place ghee and maple syrup in a saucepan and stir over a low heat until the ghee has melted
3. Add the baking soda and allow to fizz
4. Remove from the heat
5. Place flour, ginger and coconut sugar in a bowl and stir to combine
6. Add the butter mixture and stir to combine
7. Cover the mixture with a cloth and allow to sit in a warm place for 2-4 hours
8. Take a heaped teaspoon full of the mixture and roll into a ball
9. Place onto a baking tray which has been lined with non-stick baking paper
10. Bake for 12-15 minutes or until firm
11. Cool on a wire rack. The biscuits will become crisp as they cool
12. Store in an airtight container or freeze

Note: Ideally you wouldn't cook with honey as it contains delicate enzymes and antimicrobial compounds which may be damaged by heat.

Spicy pumpkin cake

Gluten Free · Vegetarian · Dairy Free · Sugar Free

Ingredients

- 1 cup peeled and cooked Jap pumpkin
- 1/2 cup of cooked, peeled golden or red beetroot
- 1/4 cup warm pure water
- 1/4 cup of Sweet Spice Blend *(p100)*
- 1 large carrot grated
- 80g maple syrup
- a good pinch of salt
- A dropper full of vanilla stevia liquid
- 1/4 cup softened ghee or coconut oil
- 1 cup *Low thiol & gluten-free* flour *(p75)*
- 1 tsp aluminium-free baking soda
- 1/2 cup activated* walnuts
- 1 cup shredded coconut
- zest of one orange or 2 drops of orange oil
- orange slices to decorate
- 2 Tbs gelatin

Method

1. Sprinkle the gelatin over the warm water, whisk with a fork to dissolve
2. Blend the vegetables, gelatin mixture, softened ghee, stevia, salt and spice together until smooth
3. Blend in the sifted flour and baking soda
4. Stir through the coconut and nuts
5. Cover the mixture with a cloth and allow to sit in a warm place for 2-4 hours
6. Pour the batter into a greased and lined spring form cake tin. Decorate with nuts or slithered almonds
7. Bake at 160°C or 320°F for 50 - 60 minutes
8. Allow to cool before moving to a cooling rack
9. Chill in the fridge to firm the cake and serve with *Whipped creamy coconut* *(p68)*

Thermomix Method

1. Place the peeled pumpkin and beets into the machine with the water. Process at speed 5 for 5 seconds. Set to Veroma (high heat) for 9 minutes, speed 2
2. Add the butter or ghee and allow to cool
3. Soften the gelatin in 1/2 cup of water and blend into the batter
4. Blend in the mixed flour, spice, salt on a low speed
5. Select reverse to mix in the coconut and nuts
6. Cook as per regular method

*For more information about why it is important to activate nuts, see page xxiv

COMPLETION TIME: 4 hours

LEVEL: Moderate

PREP: 40 min

YIELD: 8 - 10 servings

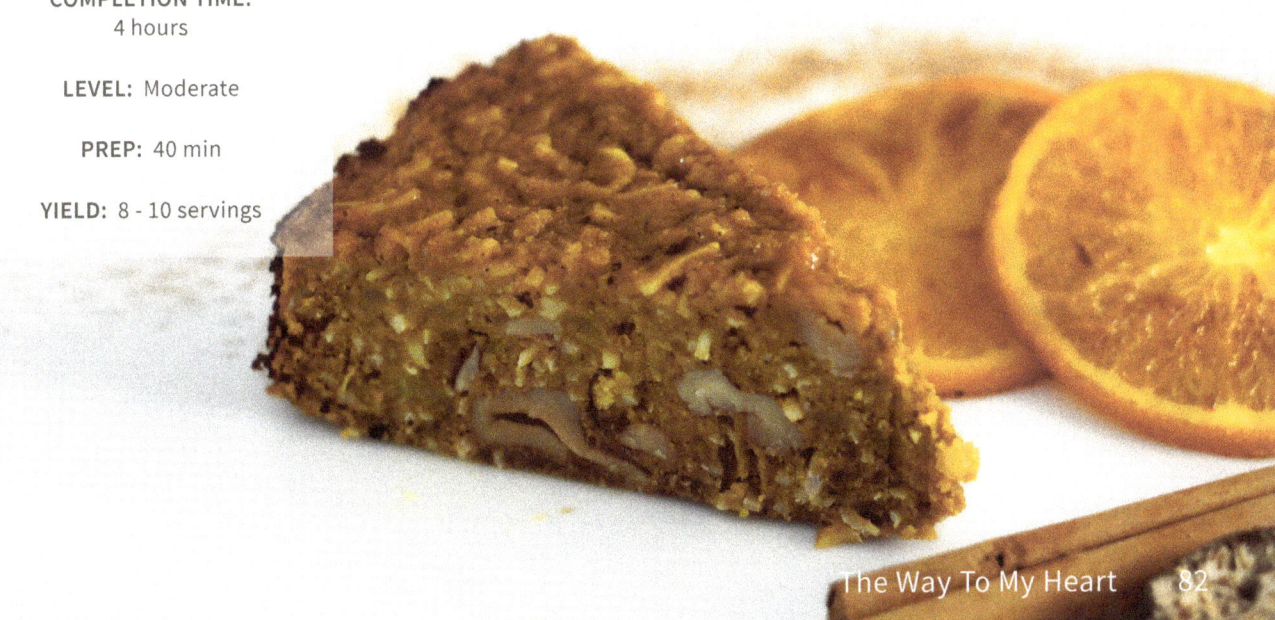

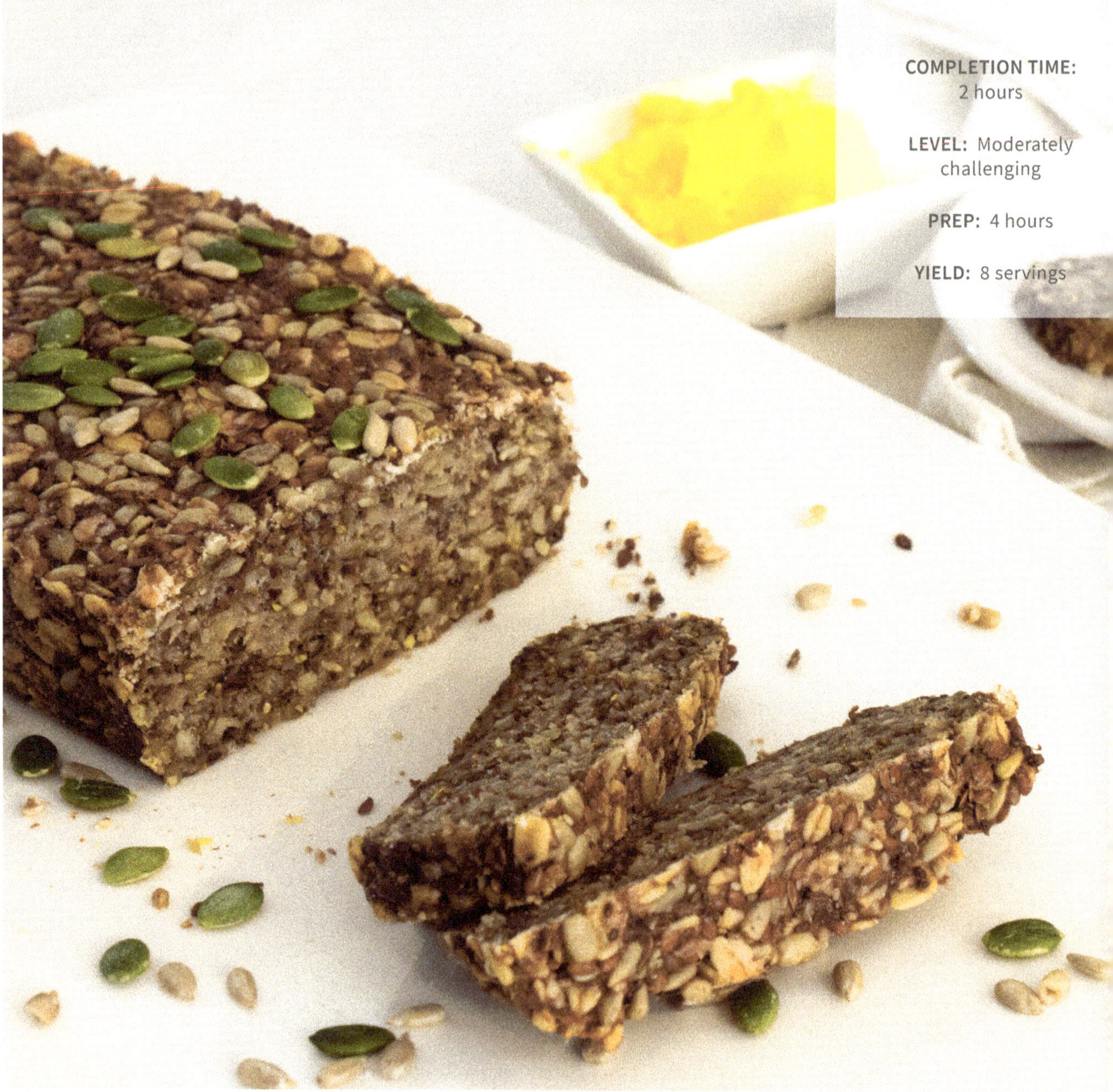

COMPLETION TIME: 2 hours

LEVEL: Moderately challenging

PREP: 4 hours

YIELD: 8 servings

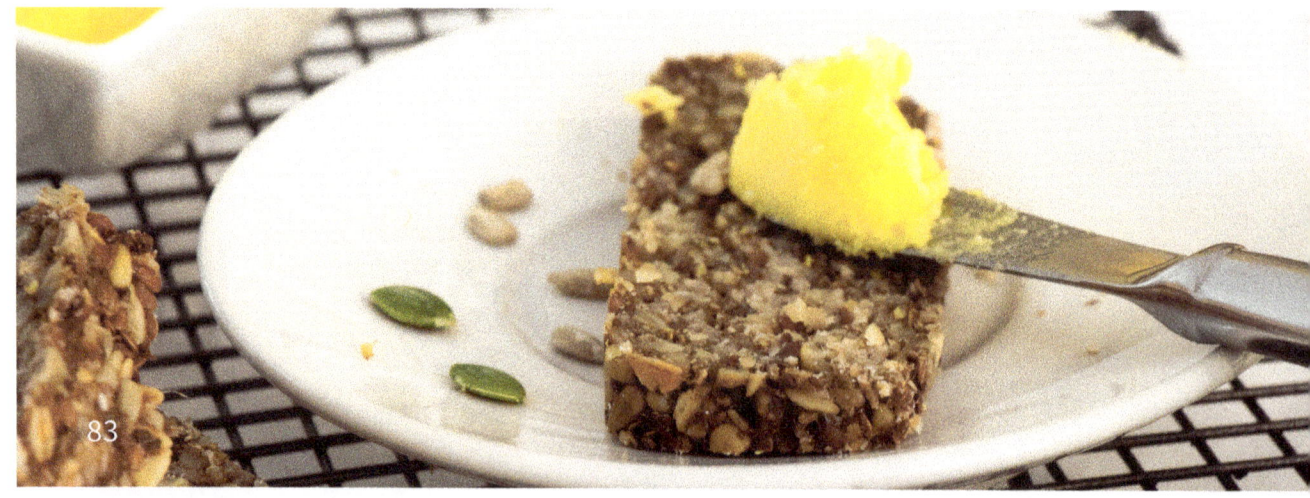

Seed loaf olive & rosemary or fig & sweet spice

Gluten Free · Vegetarian · Dairy Free · Sugar Free

Note: Kombucha is easy to make at home and makes a great live probiotic culture or starter for soaking your grains and flour. This effectively pre-digests grains reducing the enzymatic demands on the digestive system. Oregano helps to suppress yeast overgrowth commonly an issue for those with mercury toxicity. Freshly ground spices support digestive function and reduce oxidative stress resulting from heavy metal exposure.

Ingredients

- 1 cup sunflower seeds
- 1/2 cup flax seeds
- 1/2 cup almonds chopped
- 1 1/2 cups whole oat groats
- 2 Tbs chia seeds
- 2 Tbs psyllium husks
- 2 Tbs acacia fiber
- 1 tsp salt
- 1 tsp honey
- 3 Tbs ghee or melted coconut oil
- 1 cup pure water
- 1/2 cup *Kombucha (p75)*

Method

1. Preheat oven to 175°C or 350°F
2. Mix all dry ingredients in a bowl
3. Combine honey, oil, kombucha and water in a jug and add to the dry ingredients*. Mix well, if dough becomes too thick add a teaspoon of water to soften
4. Spoon mixture into a loaf pan lined with greased baking paper and smooth the top with a spatula
5. Let the pan sit at room temperature for at least 3 hours
6. Place pan in preheated oven on the middle rack and bake for about 20 minutes
7. Remove bread from pan and carefully place upside down directly onto the oven rack and bake for a further 30 - 45 minutes
8. Bread is cooked when it sounds hollow when tapped

IMPORTANT: Cool thoroughly before slicing

9. Can be sliced and frozen or kept in a sealed container in the fridge for approximately 5 days

VARIATION
Add 1/2 cup of olives and 1 Tbs dried oregano
Or 1/2 cup chopped dried figs and 1 Tbs of **Sweet spice blend** *(p100)*

*For more information about why it is important to activate nuts and seeds, see page xxiv

Spicy seed crackers

Gluten Free · Nut Free · Vegetarian · Dairy Free · Sugar Free

Ingredients

- 1 cup water
- 1/2 cup flaxseeds
- 2 Tbs chia seeds
- 3/4 cup sunflower seeds
- 1/2 cup pumpkin seds
- 1 1/2 tsp salt
- 1/2 tsp dried chilli flakes
- 1 tsp ground cumin
- pinch of pepper

Method

1. Combine the seeds, salt, chilli flakes, cumin and pepper in a bowl and add the water and mix well
2. Allow the mixture to sit for about 40 minutes or until the liquid has been absorbed*
3. Preheat oven to 150°C or 300°F
4. Spread mixture in a 1/2 cm layer onto a lined baking tray and score with a knife so that the individual crackers can be easily broken once cooked
5. Bake for 30 minutes
6. Remove tray from oven and slide the baking paper with the crackers onto a metal cooling rack. Return the rack to the oven for a further 20 - 30 minutes to bake the underside
7. Remove from oven and cool on a wire rack

Herbed seed crackers

Gluten Free · Nut Free · Vegetarian · Dairy Free · Sugar Free

Ingredients

- 1 cup water
- 1/2 cup flaxseeds
- 2 Tbs chia seeds
- 3/4 cup sunflower seeds
- 1/2 cup pumpkin seeds
- 1 tsp salt
- 1 tsp dried oregano or sage leaves
- 2 Tbs psyllium powder

Method

1. Combine the seeds, psyllium, salt and oregano in a bowl and add the water and mix well
2. Allow the mixture to sit for about 40 minutes or until the liquid has been absorbed*
3. Preheat oven to 150°C or 300°F
4. Spread mixture in a 1 cm layer onto a baking paper-lined baking tray and score with a knife so that the individual crackers can be easily broken once cooked
5. Bake for 30 minutes
6. Remove tray from oven and slide the baking paper with the crackers onto a metal cooling rack. Return the rack to the oven for a further 20 - 30 minutes to bake the underside
7. Remove from oven and cool on a wire rack

*For more information about why it is important to activate nuts and seeds, see page xxiv

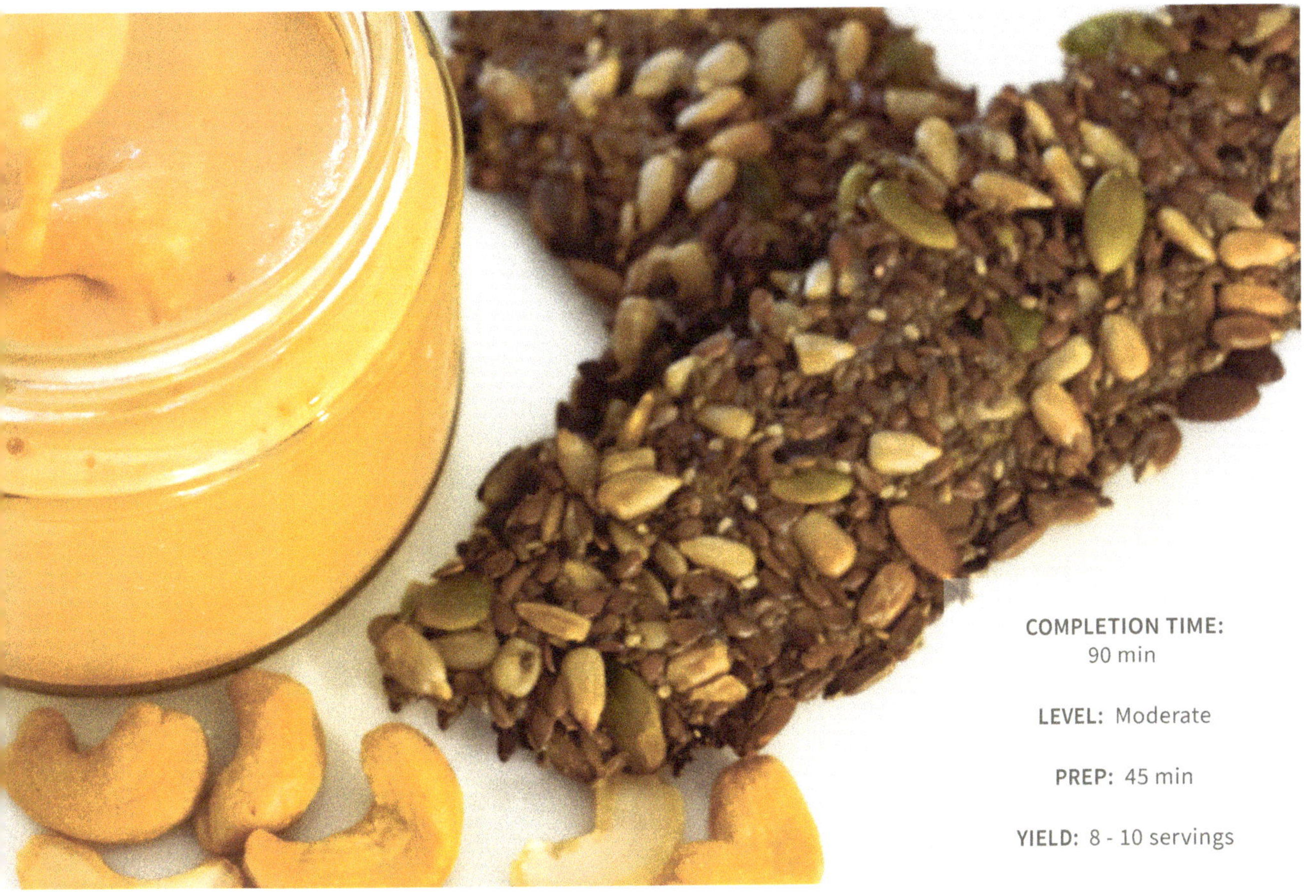

COMPLETION TIME:
90 min

LEVEL: Moderate

PREP: 45 min

YIELD: 8 - 10 servings

COMPLETION TIME:
90 min

LEVEL: Moderate

PREP: 45 min

YIELD: 8 - 10 servings

The Way To My Heart

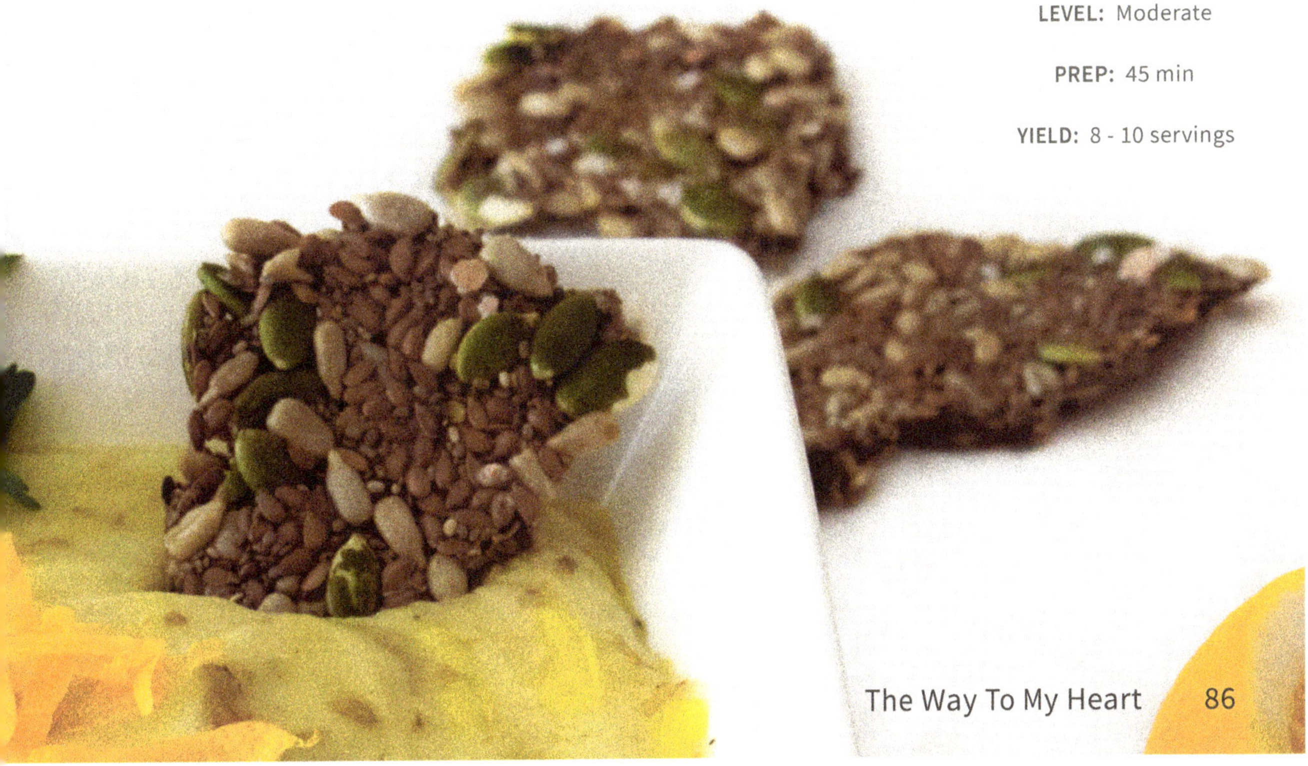

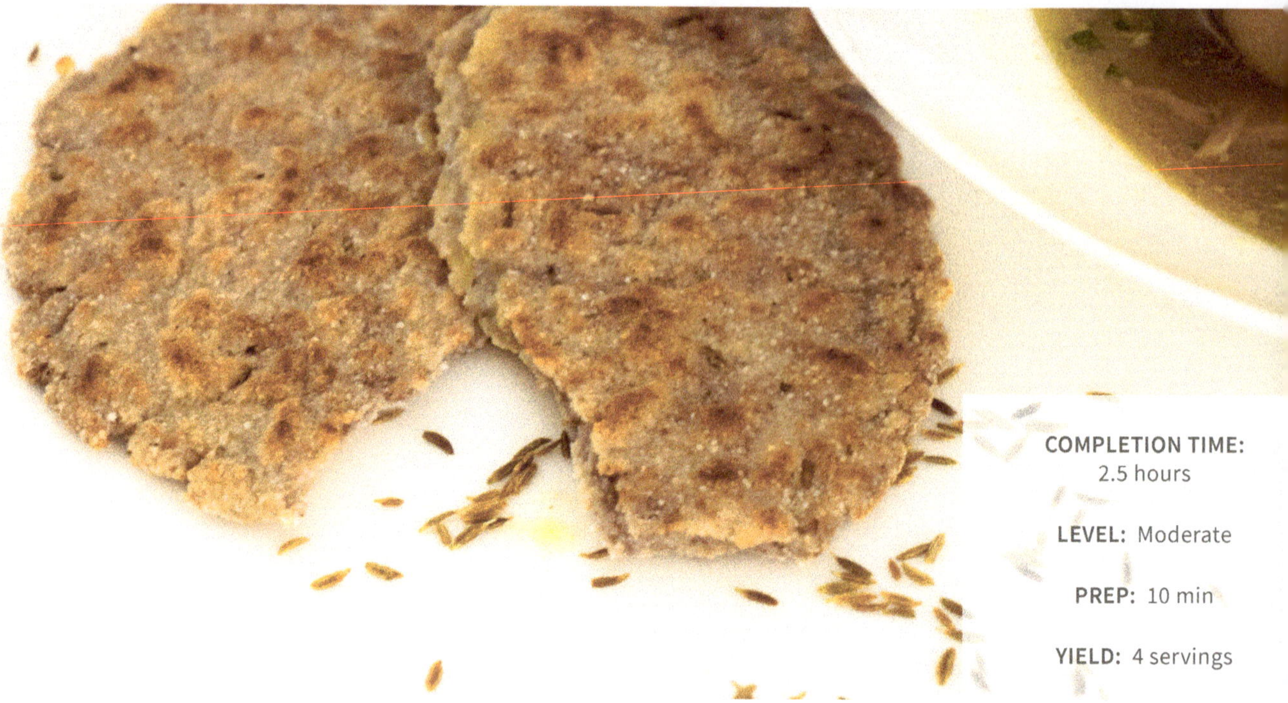

Cumin flatbread

COMPLETION TIME: 2.5 hours

LEVEL: Moderate

PREP: 10 min

YIELD: 4 servings

 Gluten Free Nut Free Vegetarian Dairy Free Sugar Free

Ingredients

2 cups whole grain sorghum flour
1 tsp ground cumin seeds
1/4 tsp salt
pinch of pepper
2 cups minus 1 Tbs hot water
1 Tbs *Kombucha (p75)*

Method

1. Combine sorghum flour, ground cumin seeds, salt and pepper in a large mixing bowl
2. Drizzle the hot water and kombucha very slowly into to the dry mix while continuously stirring the flour
3. Dough should be smooth. Divide into 6 - 8 sized balls
4. Roll each ball onto a floured surface until dough is approximately 2 mm thick
5. Cover with a cloth and allow to sit in a warm place for a couple of hours
6. Press gently using hands to achieve an even thickness
7. Cook in a hot non-stick pan for about 1 minute, brushing the top side with a little water then turn dough in the pan and cook for about 1 minute on the other side
8. Remove from pan and loosely cover with a damp cloth
9. Repeat this process for remaining dough

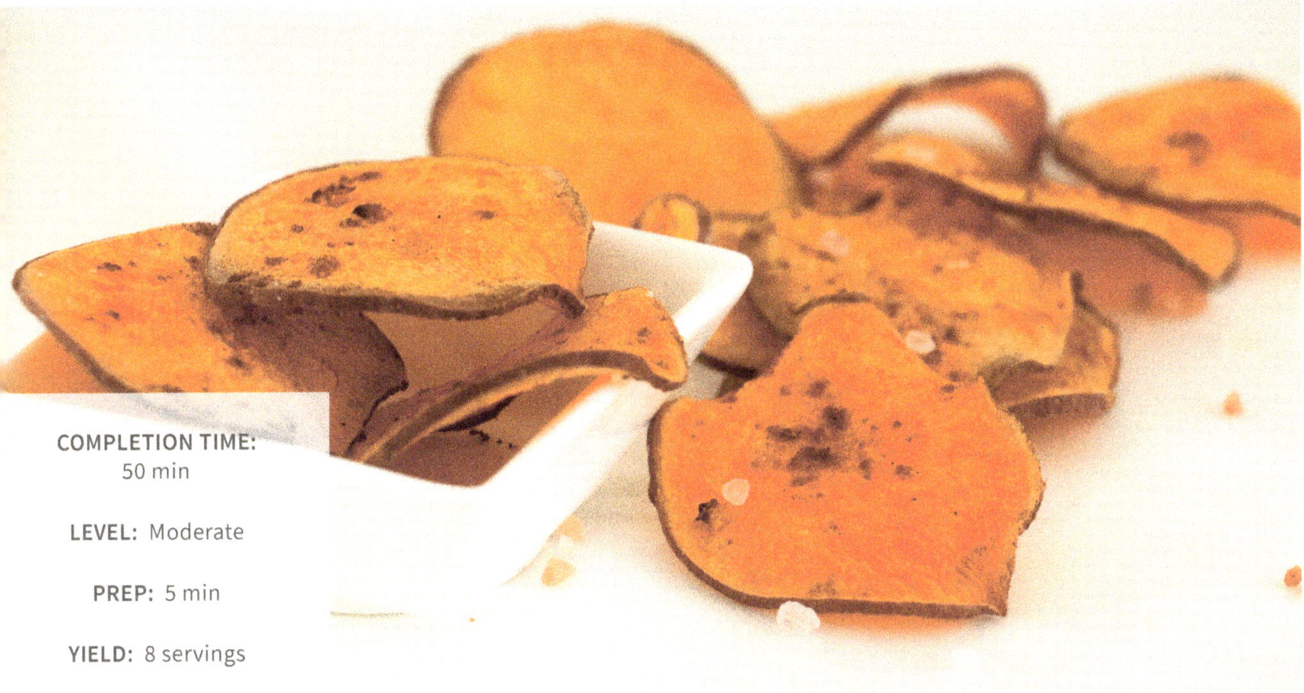

COMPLETION TIME: 50 min

LEVEL: Moderate

PREP: 5 min

YIELD: 8 servings

Chilli lime sweet potato chips

Gluten Free   Nut Free   Vegetarian   Dairy Free   Sugar Free

Ingredients

2 medium to large sweet potatoes
2 Tbs coconut oil
1 tsp very fine lime zest
3/4 teaspoon chilli powder
1/4 tsp ground cumin powder
1 tsp salt

Method

1. Preheat oven to 200°C or 392°F
2. Use a vegetable slicer or mandolin to slice sweet potatoes into thin pieces, toss well with oil and place onto a baking tray lined with baking paper
3. Sprinkle the chilli powder, cumin powder, salt and lime zest onto the sweet potato and bake for 25 - 30 minutes or until the slices are golden brown. Keep an eye on the chips taking care not to burn the thinner slices
4. Remove from oven and serve when cool

Variation: Lemon zest may be substituted for the lime zest.

Juicy kombucha _{p93}

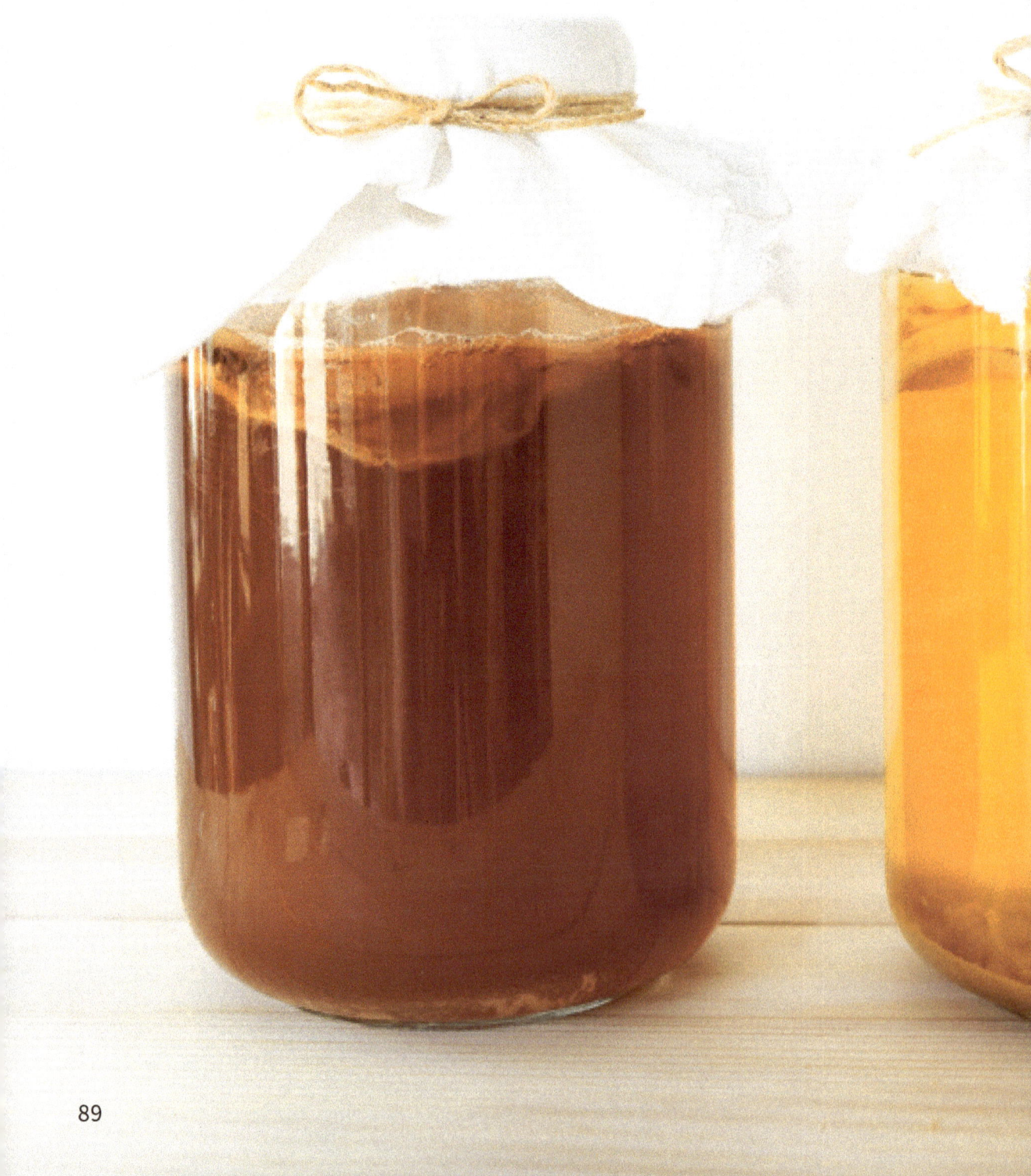

Bevvies
&
Brews
&
Condiments

Digestive tea to re-balance your gut microbes	91	Banana & almond milk smoothie	96
Chai tea	92	Nut cream fermented dip	97
Kombucha	93	Nut butter	98
Juicy Kombucha	93	Jillaine's savoury ground spice blend	99
Nut milk	95	Sweet spice blend	100

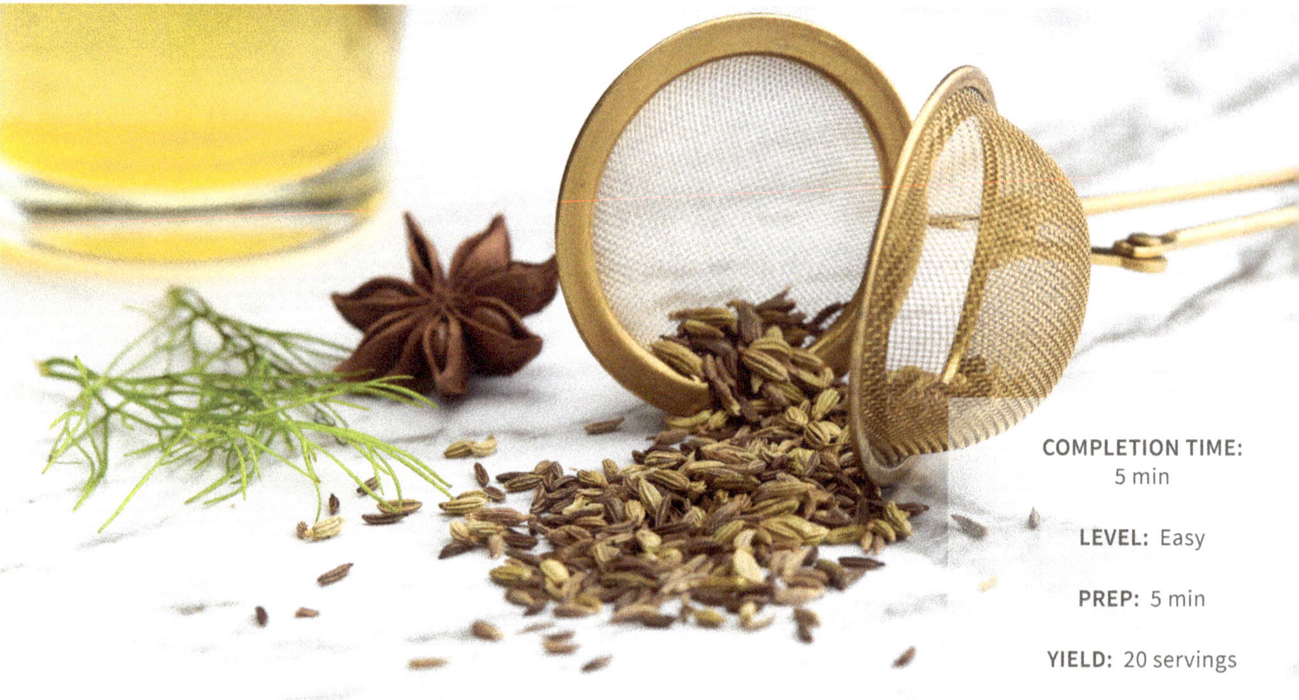

COMPLETION TIME: 5 min

LEVEL: Easy

PREP: 5 min

YIELD: 20 servings

Digestive tea to re-balance your gut microbes

Gluten Free · Nut Free · Vegetarian · Dairy Free · Sugar Free

For those with weak or sluggish digestive function Digestive Spices are gentle yet powerful in their effects- increasing bile flow, improving pancreatic and intestinal enzyme function and thus break down of foods, reducing bloat and gas production. They are known too as free radical scavengers reducing oxidative damage.

Ingredients

1/2 cup organic caraway seeds

1/2 cup organic fennel seeds

1/2 cup organic anise seeds

Method

1. Use a mortar and pestle or spice grinder to create a course blend, can be stored for one or two weeks
2. Place 1 tsp per cup into a plunger or tea ball and add boiled pure water
3. Serve with meals

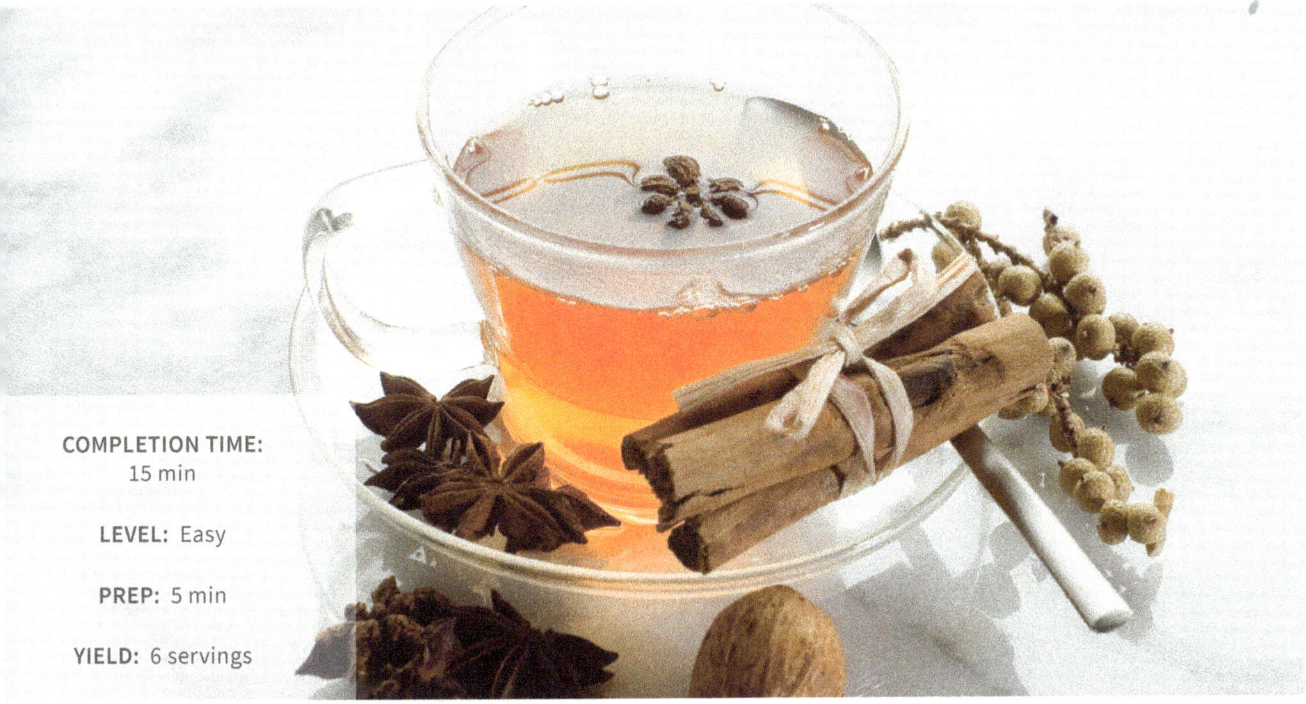

COMPLETION TIME: 15 min

LEVEL: Easy

PREP: 5 min

YIELD: 6 servings

Chai tea

Gluten Free · Nut Free · Vegetarian · Dairy Free · Sugar Free

Good quality fats such as organic ghee help to stimulate bile flow and thus detoxification. They provide cholesterol which is essential for neurological function, hormones production and immune resilience to name a few.

Ingredients

2 cinnamon sticks
2 clove buds
1 whole star anise
3 cardamom pods slightly bruised
2-3 slices of fresh ginger
1 heaped Tbs of organic tea leaves

Method

1. Place the whole spices into a 6 cup tea pot or coffee jug together with tea leaves or bags
2. Allow to steep for 3 minutes before pouring through a sieve

Option: Blend each cup of prepared tea at high speed with 2 tsp of organic ghee and / or top with Whipped creamy coconut (p68) for a creamy chai tea

Option: Use ready made Sweet spice blend (p100) together with 1 whole star anise and 2 whole cardamom pods

Kombucha

Ingredients

kombucha SCOBY (symbiotic community of bacteria and yeast) with a few Tbs of the liquid from a previous batch

1 litre boiled, pure, filtered water

6 organic tea bags

3 heaped Tbs raw organic sugar

Method

1. Place the tea bags and sugar in a large pot
2. Add the boiled water and allow to steep until cooled to body temperature
3. Place the SOBY into a 2L wide-mouthed mason or glass jar
4. Pour in the cooled tea
5. Cover loosely with a clean cloth and place a dark cupboard for around 5 days or until the SCOBY has created a new layer and the liquid has become pleasantly sour

Juicy kombucha

Using live beneficial microbes such as exist in a Kombucha SCOBY (symbiotic culture of bacteria and yeast) has multiple benefits.

They help to reduce the sugar content of fresh juice, they preserve the juice for a longer shelf life and they provide beneficial microbes for gut health and protection from recirculating heavy metals.

Ingredients

choose organic where possible

1kg green or tart Apples

1 bunch celery

2 large beets

1 x 4-5 cm piece of ginger

1 litre of ready made *Kombucha*

Method

1. Juice the apples, celery, beets and ginger and place half and half together with ready made kombucha into sealed bottles
2. Place in a warm spot for 3-4 days. You will need to 'burp' the bottles daily from around day 2 to avoid too much pressure building inside the bottles
3. Transfer the bottles to the fridge to top the fermentation process

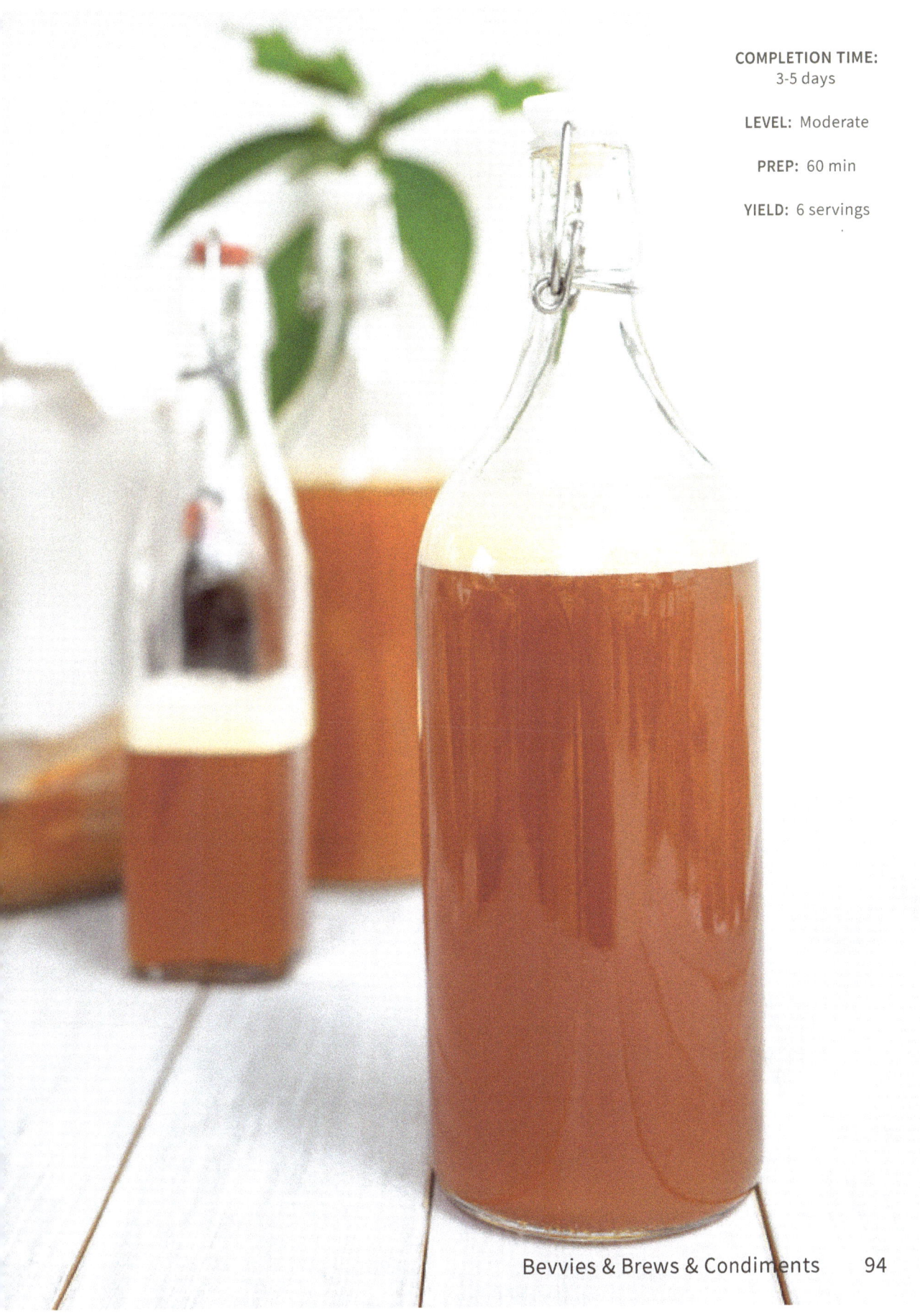

COMPLETION TIME: 3-5 days

LEVEL: Moderate

PREP: 60 min

YIELD: 6 servings

COMPLETION TIME: 30 min

LEVEL: Moderate

PREP: 6 hours

YIELD: 4 servings

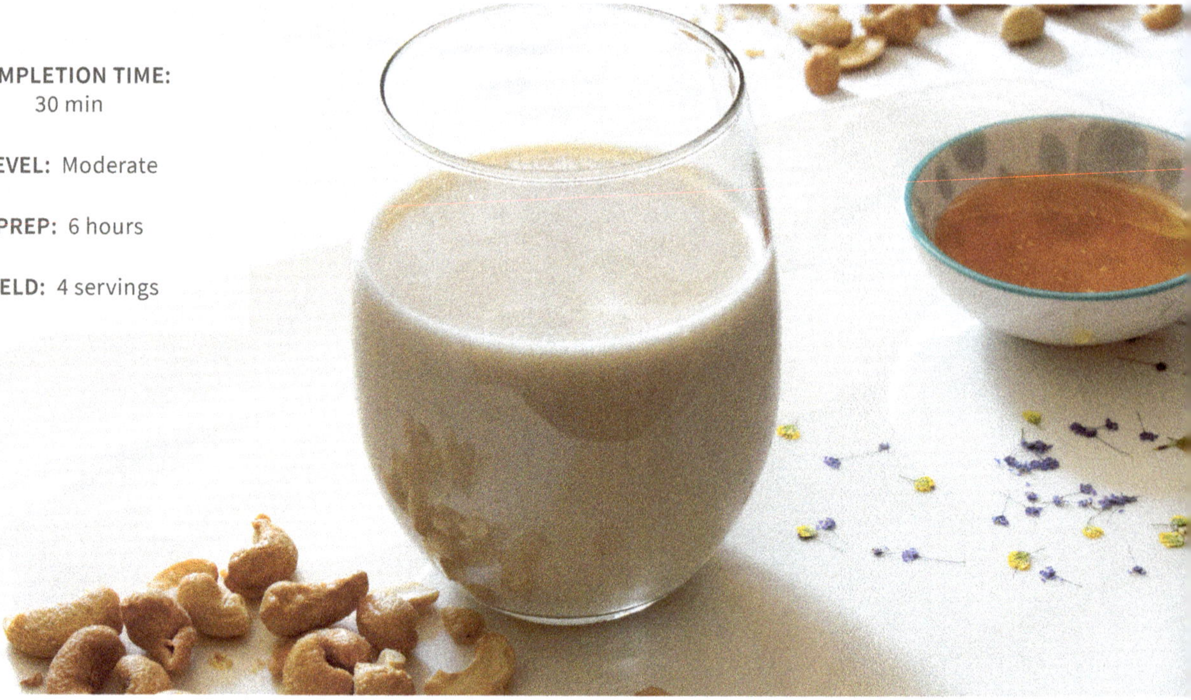

Nut milk

Gluten Free · Vegetarian · Dairy Free · Sugar Free

Ingredients

1 cup your choice of nuts or seeds- use sunflower seeds, pepita, almonds, cashews. pecans or macadamia

3 cups pure water

1 tsp salt

Optional: 1 tsp 100% vanilla, honey or maple syrup to your taste

Method

1. Place the nuts/ seeds in a large bowl and cover with water by an extra 3 cm to allow for swelling
2. Mix in the salt
3. Soak for 4-6 hours
4. Drain and rinse to discard the anti-nutrients from the nuts/ seeds
5. Place the nuts/ seeds in a food processor or blender together with the pure water, vanilla and/ or sweetener of choice
6. Blend at high speed for 2 minutes
7. Use a cheese cloth lined strainer placed over a pouring jug and strain the solids from the liquid. Gather up the bag or cloth and squeeze the remainder of liquid from the solids
8. Keep refrigerated for up to 2 days

Option: To make your own coconut milk use desiccated coconut (sulfite free) and soak in hot water for 2 hours before blending and straining.

*For more information about why it is important to activate nuts and seeds, see page xxiv

COMPLETION TIME: 10 min

LEVEL: Easy

PREP: 10 min

YIELD: 4 servings

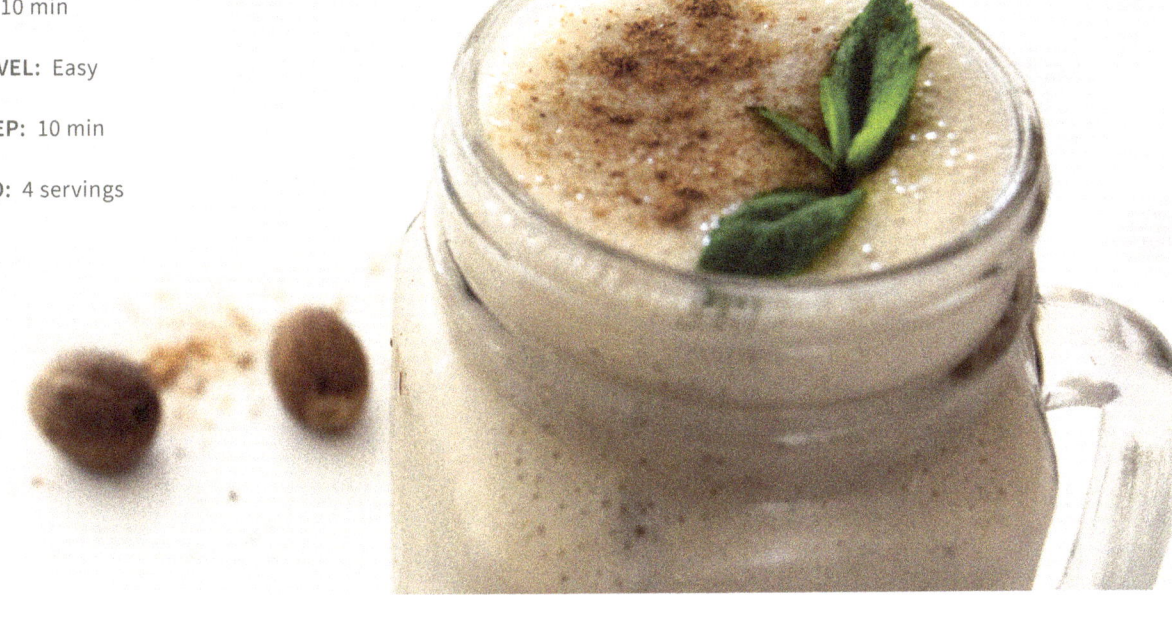

Banana & almond milk smoothie

Gluten Free   Vegetarian   Dairy Free   Sugar Free

Ingredients

1 large ripe banana

1 1/2 cups activated* almond milk (use coconut milk as a nut-free option)

2 tsp raw honey

2 ice cubes

pinch of nutmeg

Method

1. Place all ingredients into a blender and process until smooth and creamy
2. Serve immediately

Variation: Rice milk may be substituted for almond milk in the same quantity. Cinnamon may be substituted for nutmeg if desired.

*For more information about why it is important to activate nuts, see page xxiv

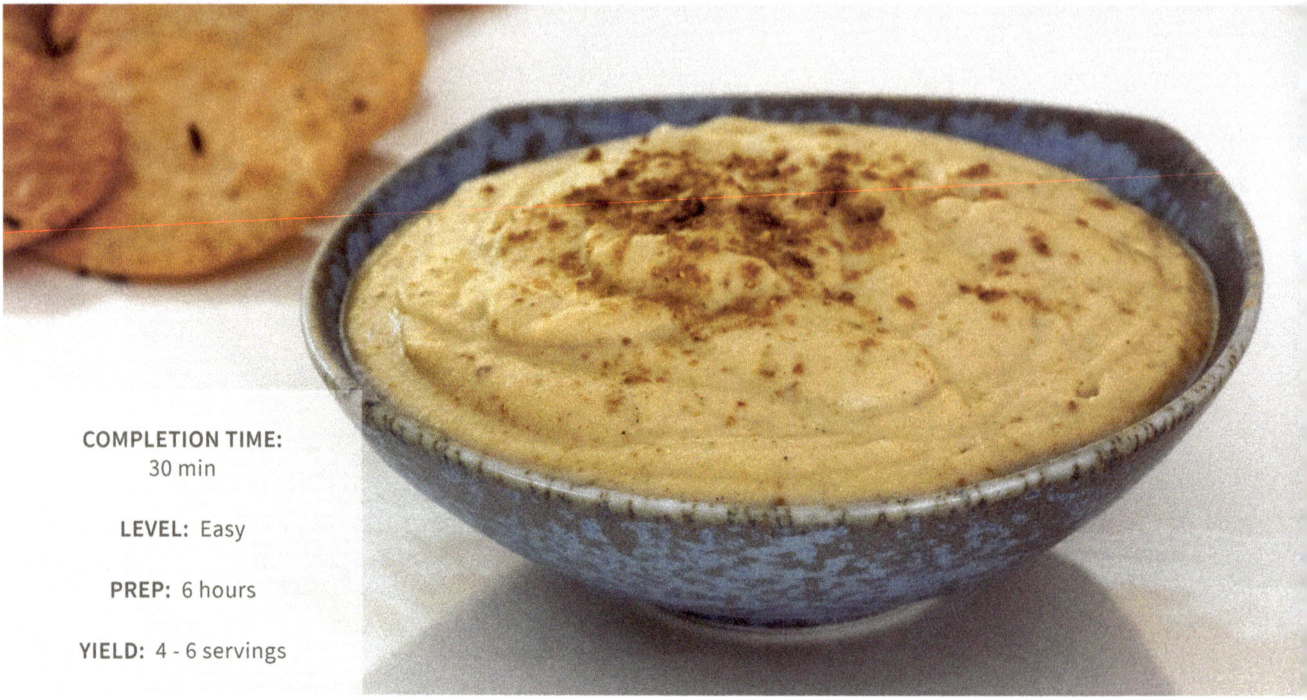

COMPLETION TIME: 30 min

LEVEL: Easy

PREP: 6 hours

YIELD: 4 - 6 servings

Nut cream fermented dip

Gluten Free Vegetarian Dairy Free Sugar Free

Cashew cream can be turned into a fermented dip. Replace 1/4 cup of water with plain or ginger and lemon Kombucha (p93), add 1/2 tsp of salt and your choice of parsley, asafoetida or spice. Place into a glass jar and cover loosely. Maintain at 43ºC for 12 hours. Seal and transfer to the fridge. Serve with seed crackers or vegetable sticks.

Ingredients

1 cup almonds or cashews (soaked for 6 hours)*

3/4 cup pure water

sweetener of your choice (optional)

Method

1. Place the soaked nuts into a blender and process to a fine meal
2. Add water and process until smooth

*For more information about why it is important to activate nuts, see page xxiv

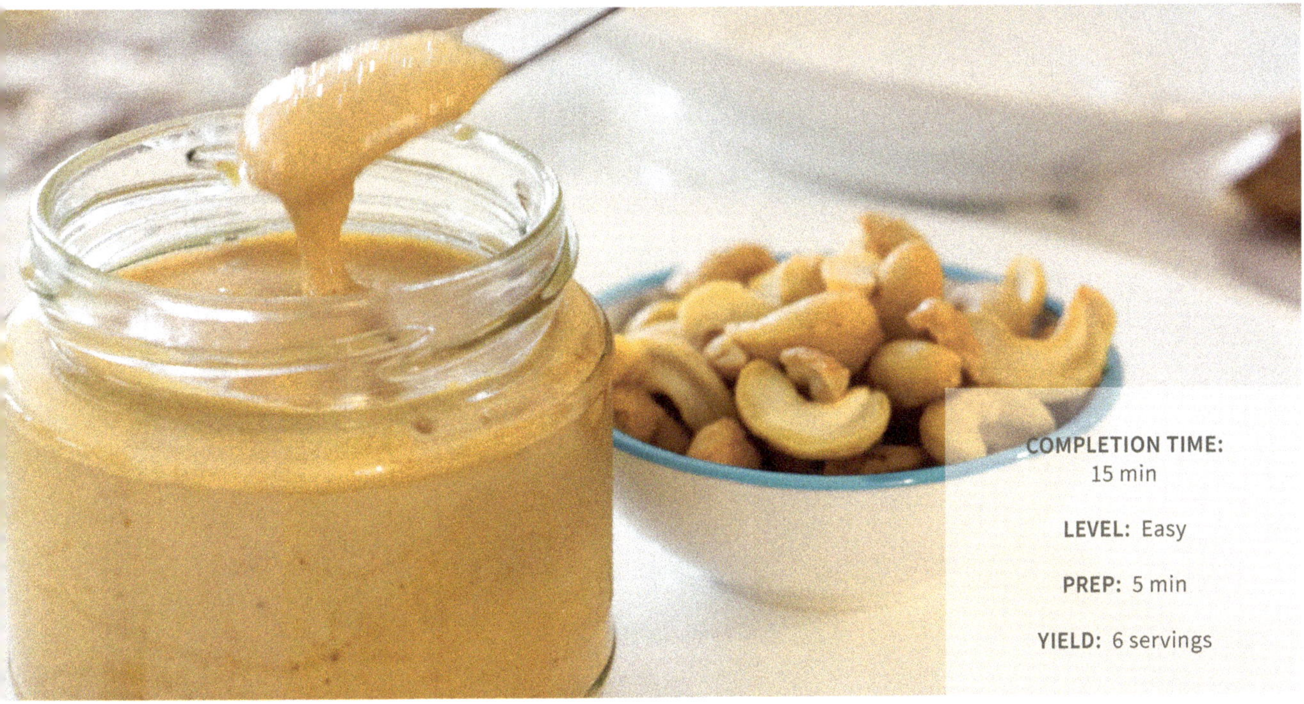

COMPLETION TIME: 15 min

LEVEL: Easy

PREP: 5 min

YIELD: 6 servings

Nut butter

 Gluten Free   Vegetarian   Dairy Free   Sugar Free

Ingredients

1 cup crispy or activated* nuts, cashews or almonds

3/4 cup melted coconut oil

1 tsp raw honey

1 tsp Himalayan salt

Method

1. Place nuts and salt into a food processor and blend to a powder
2. Add coconut oil and honey and process until smooth or to desired consistency
3. The butter will harden when refrigerated
4. Store in an airtight jar in the refrigerator

Variation: Any spice of choice may be added for extra flavour.

*For more information about why it is important to activate nuts, see page xxiv

Bevvies & Brews & Condiments

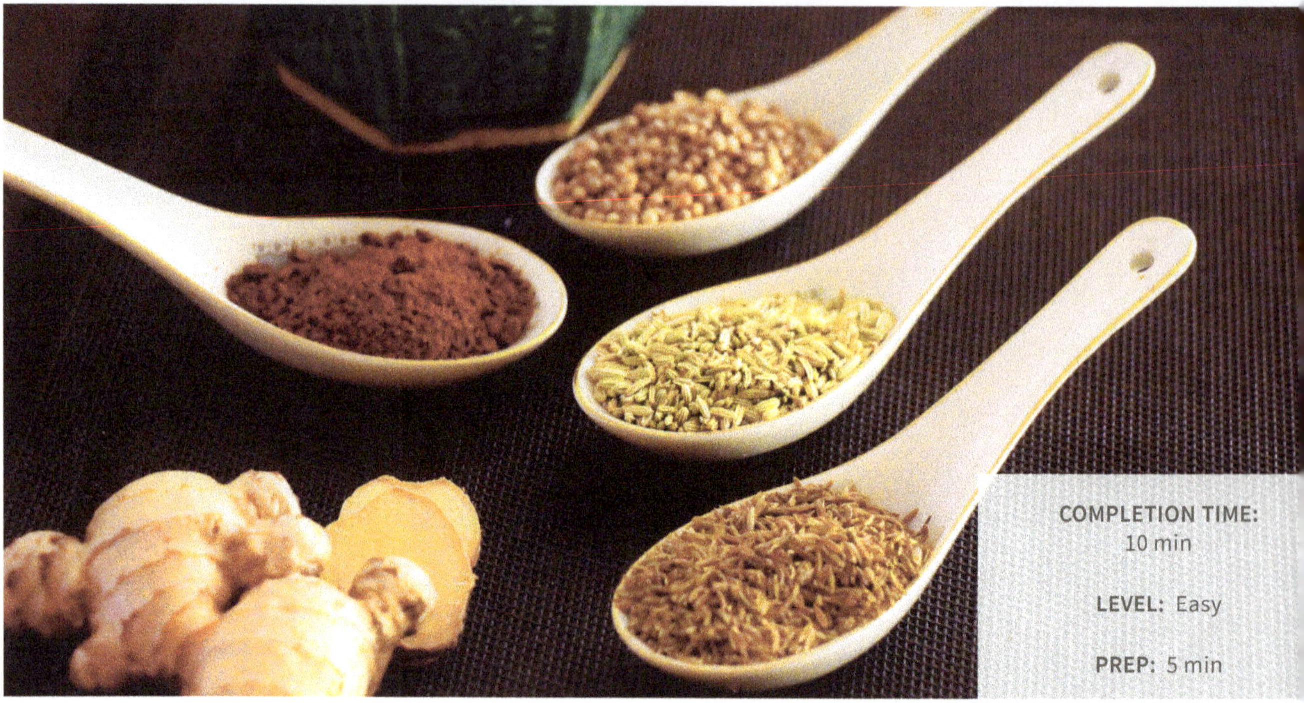

Jillaine's savoury ground spice blend

COMPLETION TIME: 10 min

LEVEL: Easy

PREP: 5 min

 Gluten Free   Nut Free   Vegetarian   Dairy Free   Sugar Free

Use this blend liberally in curries, soups, casseroles, as a marinade for meat, fish or poultry, to support digestive function and to reduce oxidative stress.

Ingredients

equal parts of the following organic spices

coriander seeds

cumin seeds

cardamom seeds

fennel seeds

ground ginger

Method

1. Use a food processor to grind to a powder
2. Store in an airtight container for up to 4 weeks

Sweet spice blend

Gluten Free   Nut Free   Vegetarian   Dairy Free   Sugar Free

Traditional Ayurvedic spices support gastric, liver and gall bladder function, also known as Phase III detoxification. Add these spices to Moroccan dishes, porridge, home made chocolate, cakes and slices to improve bile flow and thus the removal of toxins including heavy metals from the body.
I usually make up enough spice blend to last a few weeks in the kitchen. The following quantities are suitable for a family of 4 to last around 4 weeks.

Ingredients

1 cup of Cinnamon sticks or pieces
1 Tbs Ground ginger
2 Tbs Freshly grated Nutmeg
1 tsp Whole Clove buds
Add 1 Tbs of dried orange peel (optional)

Method

1. Use a food processor to grind to a powder
2. Store in an airtight container for up to 4 weeks

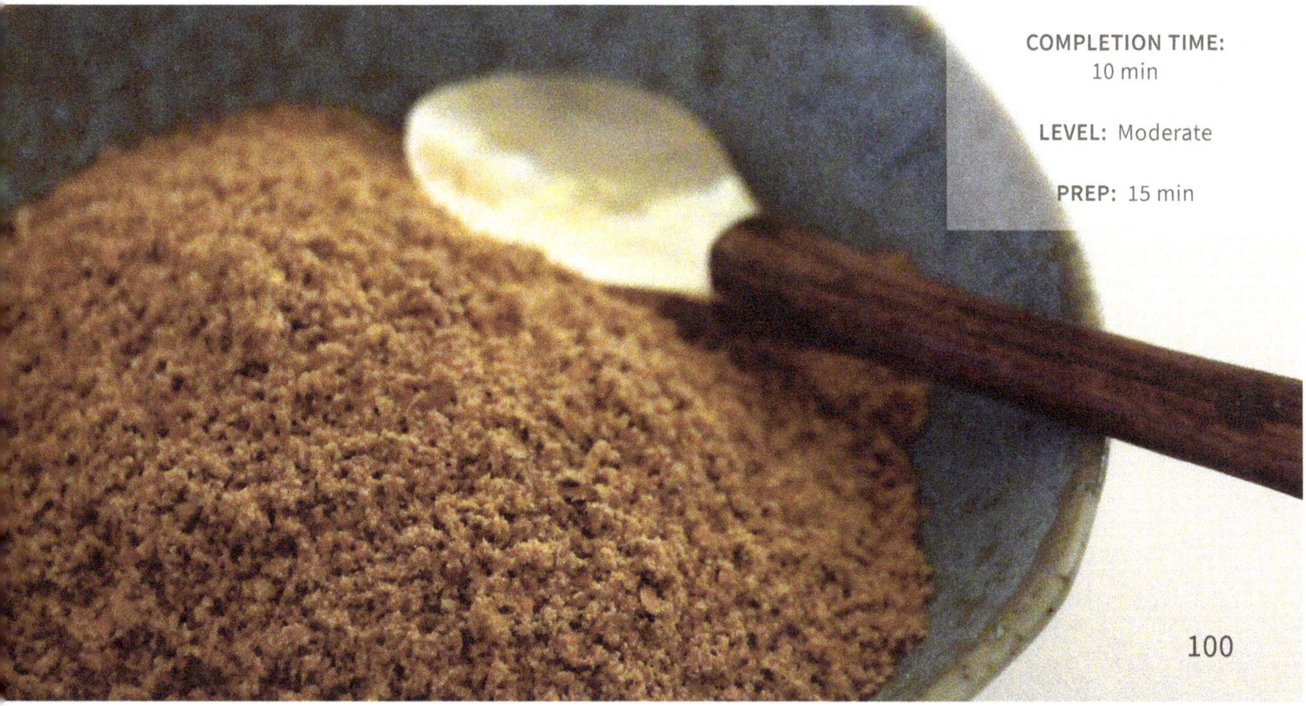

COMPLETION TIME: 10 min

LEVEL: Moderate

PREP: 15 min

Index

A
A little something on the side **13**
acacia fiber
    Seed loaf olive & rosemary or fig & sweet spice 84
allspice
    Slow cooked French rillette 55
almond
    Apple crumble 71
    Minted potato salad 17
    Nut butter 98
    Nut milk 95
    Seed loaf olive & rosemary or fig & sweet spice 84
almond, meal
    Apple crumble 71
almond, slithered
    Ginger infused rice 25
    Spicy pumpkin cake 82
anchovies
    Asian style dumplings 27
    Asian vegetable salad 18
    Italian style perch with lemon, anchovies & capers 42
    Mediterranean seafood soup 35
    Pizza with olives, anchovies & mushrooms 54
Anzac cookies 77
apple
    Apple crumble 71
    Creamy spiced porridge 11
    Juicy kombucha 93
    Muffins 75
    Spiced apple with ginger & orange zest 10
    Vegetable soup 34
apple cider vinegar
    Gluten-free banana bread 78
Apple crumble 71
apricot
    Apple crumble 71
asafoetida
    Chicken stock and bone broths 40
    Low thiol Thai curry paste 20
    Low thiol vegetable stock 16
    Mushroom pâté 7
    Organic turkey, duck or chicken liver pâté 8
    Skordalia 21
    Asian style dumplings 27
Asian vegetable salad 18
avocado
    Avocado with bacon & parsley 3
    Lemon & dill avocado 3
    Zucchini noodles with avocado pesto 22
Avocado with bacon & parsley 3

B
bacon, free-range, nitrate free
    Avocado with bacon & parsley 3
    Organic turkey, duck or chicken liver pâté 8

Baking 73
baking powder
    Banana pancakes 6
    Gluten-free banana bread 78
    Pumpkin & ginger tart 79
baking soda
    Anzac cookies 77
    Ginger snaps 81
    Gluten-free banana bread 78
    Muffins 75
    Pumpkin & ginger tart 79
    Spicy pumpkin cake 82
bamboo shoots
    Asian vegetable salad 18
banana
    Banana & almond milk smoothie 96
    Banana pancakes 6
    Gluten-free banana bread 78
Banana & almond milk smoothie 96
Banana pancakes 6
basil
    Asian vegetable salad 18
    Lemon & basil infused rice 30
    Lemongrass rice salad 43
    Mediterranean seafood soup 35
    Mushrooms with basil 9
    Pork san choy bau 44
    Roasted tomato soup 33
    Suddenly salad 62
    Thai-style fish curry 41
    Zucchini noodles with avocado pesto 22
bay leaves
    Mediterranean seafood soup 35
    Moussaka (plant based) 48
    Poultry soup 36
    Slow cooked French rillette 55
beef, fillet
    Spicy beef pilaf 52
beetroot
    Fermented veg 24
    Juicy kombucha 93
    Raw raspberry & beetroot no-cheese cake 69
    Spicy pumpkin cake 82
Beverages 89
Bevvies & brews & condiments **89**
blueberry
    Apple crumble 71
    Muffins 75
bone broth reduction .... See chicken stock & bone broth
    Asian style dumplings 27
    Not fast enough five-minute casserole 60
    Organic turkey, duck or chicken liver pâté 8
brazil nut
    Honey nut granola 5
Breakfast 1

C

Cake 82
capers
    Italian style perch with lemon, anchovies & capers 42
    Sautéed pork with lemon caper sauce 45
    Suddenly salad 62
capsicum .... *See pepper, bell*
caraway .... *See seeds*
cardamom .... *See seeds*
    Chai tea 92
    Spicy beef pilaf 52
carrot
    Asian style dumplings 27
    Asian vegetable salad 18
    Carrots with honey orange glaze 26
    Chicken stock and bone broths 40
    Fermented veg 24
    Low thiol vegetable stock 16
    Moussaka (plant based) 48
    Poultry soup 36
    Roast vegetable medley 50
    Root vegetables roasted with hazelnuts 49
    Spicy pumpkin cake 82
    Vegetable soup 34
Carrots with honey orange glaze 26
cashew
    Muffins 75
    Nut butter 98
    Nut cream fermented dip 97
    Nut milk 95
Cashew custard 68
cassava powder
    Sautéed pork with lemon caper sauce 45
casserole 60
celery
    Asian style dumplings 27
    Chicken stock and bone broths 40
    Juicy kombucha 93
    Low thiol vegetable stock 16
    Poultry soup 36
    Vegetable soup 34
Chai tea 92
Chai tea chia pudding 12
chicken
    Right now roast 63
    Slow cooked French rillette 55
Chicken stock and bone broths 40
chicken, duck or turkey
    Poultry soup 36
chicken, frame
    Chicken stock and bone broths 40
chicken, skinless breast
    Coconut poached chicken with lime 51
chilli
    Coconut poached chicken with lime 51
    Lemongrass rice salad 43
    Pork san choy bau 44
    Roasted tomato soup 33
    Spiced roast duck 53
    Vegetable soup 34
Chilli lime sweet potato chips 88

chilli, flakes
    Spicy seed crackers 85
chilli, powder
    Chilli lime sweet potato chips 88
cinnamon
    Chai tea 92
    Lemon spice gummies 72
    Spicy beef pilaf 52
    Sweet spice blend 100
clove
    Chai tea 92
    Lemon spice gummies 72
    Sweet spice blend 100
coconut aminos
    Asian vegetable salad 18
    Pork san choy bau 44
    Vegetable soup 34
coconut cream
    Pumpkin & ginger tart 79
    I could cry - creamy soup 59
    Raw raspberry & beetroot no-cheese cake 69
coconut milk .... *See milk, coconut*
Coconut poached chicken with lime 51
coconut, shredded
    Anzac cookies 77
    Apple crumble 71
    Honey nut granola 5
    Spicy pumpkin cake 82
corn starch
    Asian style dumplings 27
    Thai-style fish curry 41
Creamy spiced porridge 11
cucumber
    Asian vegetable salad 18
    Minted potato salad 17
cumin .... *See seeds*
Cumin flatbread 87
curry 20, 41, 64

D

dates
    Creamy spiced porridge 11
    Muffins 75
    Raw raspberry & beetroot no-cheese cake 69
Dessert 65
Digestive tea 91
dill
    Lemon & dill avocado 3
    Pickled wild salmon 56
duck
    Spiced roast duck 53
duck fat
    Mushroom pâté 7
    Organic turkey, duck or chicken liver pâté 8
    Sautéed pork with lemon caper sauce 45

E

eggplant
    Moussaka (plant based) 48
    Roast vegetable medley 50

essential oil, clove
    Lemon spice gummies 72
essential oil, lemon
    Lemon spice gummies 72
essential oil, lemongrass
    Lemon spice gummies 72

F

fennel .... *See seeds*
fennel bulb
    Low thiol vegetable stock 16
ferment 6, 24, 44, 97
Fermented veg 24
fish
    Italian style perch with lemon, anchovies & capers 42
    Mediterranean seafood soup 35
    Pickled wild salmon 56
    Resuscitating Thai curry 64
    Thai-style fish curry 41
fish sauce
    Asian vegetable salad 18
    Pork san choy bau 44
    Thai-style fish curry 41
five spice
    Pork san choy bau 44
flour, arrowroot
    Pizza with olives, anchovies & mushrooms 54
flour, banana
    Low thiol & gluten-free flour 75
flour, coconut
    Pizza with olives, anchovies & mushrooms 54
flour, gluten-free
    Ginger snaps 81
    Gluten-free banana bread 78
    Pumpkin & ginger tart 79
    Spicy pumpkin cake 82
flour, oat
    Banana pancakes 6
flour, rice
    Asian style dumplings 27
    Banana pancakes 6
flour, sorghum
    Anzac cookies 77
    Cumin flatbread 87
    Low thiol & gluten-free flour 75
flour, tapioca
    Asian style dumplings 27
    Cashew custard 68
    Low thiol & gluten-free flour 75
    Moussaka (plant based) 48
    Pizza with olives, anchovies & mushrooms 54
flour, teff
    Low thiol & gluten-free flour 75

G

gelatin
    Lemon spice gummies 72
    Spicy pumpkin cake 82
ghee
    Anzac cookies 77

Apple crumble 71
Asian style dumplings 27
Avocado with bacon & parsley 3
Banana pancakes 6
Carrots with honey orange glaze 26
Honey nut granola 5
Italian style perch with lemon, anchovies & capers 42
Jillaine's raw honey drizzle 68
Mushrooms with basil 9
Not fast enough five-minute casserole 60
Pork san choy bau 44
Pumpkin & ginger tart 79
Right now roast 63
Roast vegetable medley 50
Root vegetables roasted with hazelnuts 49
Sautéed pork with lemon caper sauce 45
Spicy beef pilaf 52
Spicy pumpkin cake 82
Thai-style fish curry 41
ginger
    Asian style dumplings 27
    Chai tea 92
    Coconut poached chicken with lime 51
    Fermented veg 24
    Ginger infused rice 25
    Ginger snaps 81
    Juicy kombucha 93
    Lemon spice gummies 72
    Low thiol Thai curry paste 20
    Pumpkin & ginger tart 79
    Spiced apple with ginger & orange zest 10
Ginger infused rice 25
Ginger snaps 81
ginger, ground
    Jillaine's savoury ground spice blend 99
    Sweet spice blend 100
Gluten-free banana bread 78
gluten-free flour .... *See flour, gluten-free*
goose fat
    Mushroom pâté 7
    Organic turkey, duck or chicken liver pâté ... 8
    Sautéed pork with lemon caper sauce 45

H

hake
    Mediterranean seafood soup 35
hazelnut
    Honey nut granola 5
    Root vegetables roasted with hazelnuts 49
Herbed seed crackers 85
herbs
    Herbed seed crackers 85
    Not fast enough five-minute casserole 60
honey
    Anzac cookies 77
    Banana & almond milk smoothie 96
    Banana pancakes 6
    Carrots with honey orange glaze 26
    Chai tea chia pudding 12
    Creamy spiced porridge 11
    Ginger snaps 81

Honey nut granola 5
Jillaine's raw honey drizzle 68
Lemon spice gummies 72
Muffins 75
Nut butter 98
Nut milk 95
Pickled wild salmon 56
Seed loaf olive & rosemary or fig & sweet spice 84
Honey nut granola 5

I
I could cry - creamy soup 59
I'm just too tired to cook **57**
Italian style perch with lemon, anchovies & capers 42

J
Jillaine's raw honey drizzle 68
Jillaine's savoury ground spice blend
   Spiced roast duck 53
Jillaine's savoury ground spice blend 99
Juicy kombucha 93

K
kaffir lime leaf
   Asian vegetable salad 18
   Lemongrass rice salad 43
kombucha
   Banana pancakes 6
   Fermented veg 24
   Juicy kombucha 93
   Muffins 75
   Pickled wild salmon 56
   Seed loaf olive & rosemary or fig & sweet spice 84
Kombucha 93
kombucha SCOBY
   Kombucha 93

L
lemon
   Coconut poached chicken with lime 51
   Italian style perch with lemon, anchovies & capers 42
   Lemon & basil infused rice 30
   Lemon & dill avocado 3
   Lemon spice gummies 72
   Mushroom pâté 7
   Pickled wild salmon 56
   Pork san choy bau 44
   Poultry soup 36
   Raw raspberry & beetroot no-cheese cake 69
   Sautéed pork with lemon caper sauce 45
   Skordalia 21
   Spiced apple with ginger & orange zest 10
   Suddenly salad 62
   Zucchini noodles with avocado pesto 22
Lemon & basil infused rice 30
Lemon & dill avocado 3
Lemon spice gummies 72
lemon, preserved
   Mediterranean seafood soup 35
lemon, zest

Lemon & basil infused rice 30
lemongrass
   Lemongrass rice salad 43
   Low thiol Thai curry paste 20
Lemongrass rice salad 43
lettuce
   Suddenly salad 62
lettuce, butter
   Asian vegetable salad 18
lettuce, cos
   Pork san choy bau 44
lime, juice
   Asian vegetable salad 18
   Coconut poached chicken with lime 51
   Lemon & dill avocado 3
   Lemongrass rice salad 43
   Spiced roast duck 53
   Thai-style fish curry 41
lime, zest
   Chilli lime sweet potato chips 88
linseed .... *See seeds, flaxseeds*
livers, organic
   Organic turkey, duck or chicken liver pâté 8
Low thiol & gluten-free flour 75
Low thiol Thai curry paste 20
Low thiol vegetable stock 16

M
Main course 37
maple syrup
   Cashew custard 68
   Chai tea chia pudding 12
   Creamy spiced porridge 11
   Ginger snaps 81
   Muffins 75
   Nut milk 95
   Raw raspberry & beetroot no-cheese cake 69
   Spicy pumpkin cake 82
   Whipped creamy coconut 68
meat, chicken, pork, beef or lamb
   Lemongrass rice salad 43
meat, rabbit or chicken
   Slow cooked French rillette 55
meat, roasted
   Not fast enough five-minute casserole 60
   Resuscitating Thai curry 64
Mediterranean seafood soup 35
milk .... *See milk, almond, coconut or nut*
milk, almond
   Banana & almond milk smoothie 96
   Banana pancakes 6
   Creamy spiced porridge 11
   Moussaka (plant based) 48
   Roasted tomato soup 33
milk, cashew
   Cashew custard 68
milk, coconut
   Banana pancakes 6
   Coconut poached chicken with lime 51
   Creamy spiced porridge 11
   Moussaka (plant based) 48

Resuscitating Thai curry 64
Roasted tomato soup 33
Thai-style fish curry 41
Whipped creamy coconut 68
millet
Creamy spiced porridge 11
mint
Asian vegetable salad 18
Lemon & dill avocado 3
Minted potato salad 17
Pork san choy bau 44
Spicy beef pilaf 52
Minted potato salad 17
Moussaka (plant based) 48
Muffins 75
mushroom
Asian style dumplings 27
Avocado with bacon & parsley 3
Chicken stock and bone broths 40
Moussaka (plant based) 48
Mushroom pâté 7
Mushrooms with basil 9
Pizza with olives, anchovies & mushrooms 54
Poultry soup 36
Mushroom pâté 7
Mushrooms with basil 9
mushroom, dried
Mushroom pâté 7

N

Not fast enough five-minute casserole 60
nut butter
Honey nut granola 5
Mushroom pâté 7
Nut butter 98
nut cream
Pumpkin & ginger tart 79
Nut cream fermented dip 97
Nut milk 95
nutmeg
Asian style dumplings 27
Banana & almond milk smoothie 96
Moussaka (plant based) 48
Mushroom pâté 7
Slow cooked French rillette 55
Sweet spice blend 100
nuts
Nut butter 98
Nut cream fermented dip 97
Nut milk 95
Raw raspberry & beetroot no-cheese cake 69

O

oats, rolled
Anzac cookies 77
Honey nut granola 5
Muffins 75
oats, whole groats
Creamy spiced porridge 11
Seed loaf olive & rosemary or fig & sweet spice 84

oil, avocado
Zucchini noodles with avocado pesto 22
oil, coconut
Banana pancakes 6
Chilli lime sweet potato chips 88
Gluten-free banana bread 78
Lemongrass rice salad 43
Nut butter 98
Raw raspberry & beetroot no-cheese cake 69
Seed loaf olive & rosemary or fig & sweet spice 84
Thai-style fish curry 41
oil, hazelnut
Lemon & dill avocado 3
Minted potato salad 17
Root vegetables roasted with hazelnuts 49
oil, olive
Low thiol Thai curry paste 20
Moussaka (plant based) 48
Mushroom pâté 7
Resuscitating Thai curry 64
Right now roast 63
Roasted tomato soup 33
Skordalia 21
Spicy beef pilaf 52
Suddenly salad 62
oil, sesame
Asian vegetable salad 18
Pork san choy bau 44
Spiced roast duck 53
oil, walnut
Lemon & dill avocado 3
Minted potato salad 17
olives
Mediterranean seafood soup 35
Pizza with olives, anchovies & mushrooms 54
Suddenly salad 62
orange
Spiced roast duck 53
orange juice
Carrots with honey orange glaze 26
orange, oil
Spicy pumpkin cake 82
orange, peel
Sweet spice blend 100
orange, zest
Spiced apple with ginger & orange zest 10
oregano
Roasted tomato soup 33
Vegetable soup 34
Organic turkey, duck or chicken liver pâté 8

P

pancake 6
parsley
Avocado with bacon & parsley 3
Carrots with honey orange glaze 26
Low thiol vegetable stock 16
Moussaka (plant based) 48
Mushroom pâté 7
Organic turkey, duck or chicken liver pâté 8
Poultry soup 36

Root vegetables roasted with hazelnuts	49
Sautéed pork with lemon caper sauce	45
Skordalia	21
Suddenly salad	62
Vegetable soup	34

parsnip
Low thiol vegetable stock	16
Roast vegetable medley	50
Root vegetables roasted with hazelnuts	49
Vegetable soup	34

pâté	7, 8

peanuts
Asian vegetable salad	18

pecan, nuts
Creamy spiced porridge	11

pepitas .... *See seeds, pumpkin*

pepper, bell .... *See capsicum*
Asian vegetable salad	18
Low thiol Thai curry paste	20
Mediterranean seafood soup	35
Roast vegetable medley	50
Roasted tomato soup	33
Thai-style fish curry	41
Vegetable soup	34

perch fillets
Italian style perch with lemon, anchovies & capers	42

Pickled wild salmon	56

pistachio
Zucchini noodles with avocado pesto	22

Pizza with olives, anchovies & mushrooms	54

pomegranate molasses
Spiced apple with ginger & orange zest	10

pork
Pork san choy bau	44
Sautéed pork with lemon caper sauce	45
Slow cooked French rillette	55

Pork san choy bau	44

potato
Minted potato salad	17
Moussaka (plant based)	48
Root vegetables roasted with hazelnuts	49
Skordalia	21
Thai-style fish curry	41
Vegetable soup	34

Poultry soup	36

psyllium
Herbed seed crackers	85
Honey nut granola	5
Seed loaf olive & rosemary or fig & sweet spice	84

pumpkin
Pumpkin & ginger tart	79
Roast vegetable medley	50
Spiced roast pumpkin	29
Spicy pumpkin cake	82
Thai-style fish curry	41
Vegetable soup	34

Pumpkin & ginger tart	79

Q

Quick easy solutions	57

R

raisins
Apple crumble	71

rapadura .... *See sugar*

raspberries
Muffins	75
Raw raspberry & beetroot no-cheese cake	69

Raw raspberry & beetroot no-cheese cake	69
Resuscitating Thai curry	64

rice
Lemongrass rice salad	43

rice, basmati
Ginger infused rice	25
Lemon & basil infused rice	30
Spicy beef pilaf	52

rice, red
Creamy spiced porridge	11
Thai-style fish curry	41

rice, black
Creamy spiced porridge	11

Right now roast	63
RISE and SHINE the morning's fine	***1***
Roast vegetable medley	50
Roasted tomato soup	33
Root vegetables roasted with hazelnuts	49

rosemary
Italian style perch with lemon, anchovies & capers	42
Low thiol vegetable stock	16
Roast vegetable medley	50

S

saffron
Mediterranean seafood soup	35
Spicy beef pilaf	52

sage
Chicken stock and bone broths	40
Spiced roast duck	53

salad	17, 18, 43, 62
Sautéed pork with lemon caper sauce	45
Seed loaf olive & rosemary or fig & sweet spice	84

seeds, anise
Digestive tea	91

seeds, caraway
Digestive tea	91
Fermented veg	24

seeds, cardamom
Jillaine's savoury ground spice blend	99

seeds, chia
Chai tea chia pudding	12
Herbed seed crackers	85
Seed loaf olive & rosemary or fig & sweet spice	84
Spicy seed crackers	85

seeds, coriander
Jillaine's savoury ground spice blend	99

seeds, cumin
Asian style dumplings	27
Chilli lime sweet potato chips	88
Cumin flatbread	87
Jillaine's savoury ground spice blend	99
Low thiol Thai curry paste	20

Spicy beef pilaf 52
Spicy seed crackers 85
seeds, dill
   Fermented veg 24
seeds, fennel
   Digestive tea 91
   Jillaine's savoury ground spice blend 99
   Spicy beef pilaf 52
seeds, flaxseeds
   Herbed seed crackers 85
   Seed loaf olive & rosemary or fig & sweet spice 84
   Spicy seed crackers 85
seeds, pumpkin
   Herbed seed crackers 85
   Nut milk 95
   Spicy seed crackers 85
seeds, sunflower
   Herbed seed crackers 85
   Nut milk 95
   Seed loaf olive & rosemary or fig & sweet spice 84
   Spicy seed crackers 85
side dishes 13
Skordalia 21
Slow cooked French rillette 55
sorghum ..... See flour
sorghum, whole
   Creamy spiced porridge 11
soup 33, 34, 35, 36, 59
Spiced apple with ginger & orange zest 10
Spiced roast duck 53
Spiced roast pumpkin 29
Spicy beef pilaf 52
Spicy pumpkin cake 82
Spicy seed crackers 85
Squash, summer ..... See pumpkin
star anise
   Chai tea 92
stevia, vanilla
   Spicy pumpkin cake 82
stock See also chicken stock & bone broth
   Coconut poached chicken with lime 51
   Lemon & basil infused rice 30
   Mediterranean seafood soup 35
   Moussaka (plant based) 48
   Mushrooms with basil 9
   Roasted tomato soup 33
   Sautéed pork with lemon caper sauce 45
   Spicy beef pilaf 52
   Vegetable soup 34
Suddenly salad 62
sugar
   Kombucha 93
sugar, rapadura or coconut
   Anzac cookies 77
   Apple crumble 71
   Ginger snaps 81
   Gluten-free banana bread 78
   Lemongrass rice salad 43
   Pumpkin & ginger tart 79
   Spiced roast duck 53
sweet potato
   Chilli lime sweet potato chips 88

Low thiol vegetable stock 16
Pizza with olives, anchovies & mushrooms 54
Root vegetables roasted with hazelnuts 49
sweet spice blend
   Apple crumble 71
   Banana pancakes 6
   Creamy spiced porridge 11
   Ginger snaps 81
   Gluten-free banana bread 78
   Jillaine's raw honey drizzle 68
   Muffins 75
   Pumpkin & ginger tart 79
   Raw raspberry & beetroot no-cheese cake 69
   Spicy pumpkin cake 82
Sweet spice blend 100

T
tapioca starch ..... See flour, tapioca
tea
   Chai tea 92
   Kombucha 93
teff ..... See flour
Thai basil
   Low thiol Thai curry paste 20
Thai Curry Paste
   Resuscitating Thai curry 64
   Thai-style fish curry 41
Thai-style fish curry 41
The main attraction ***37***
The way to my heart - Gluten-free Baking ***73***
thyme
   Low thiol vegetable stock 16
   Mediterranean seafood soup 35
   Moussaka (plant based) 48
   Mushroom pâté 7
   Organic turkey, duck or chicken liver pâté 8
   Pizza with olives, anchovies & mushrooms 54
   Poultry soup 36
   Right now roast 63
   Roast vegetable medley 50
   Slow cooked French rillette 55
   Vegetable soup 34
tomato
   Asian vegetable salad 18
   Mediterranean seafood soup 35
   Moussaka (plant based) 48
   Pizza with olives, anchovies & mushrooms 54
   Roasted tomato soup 33
   Suddenly salad 62

V
vanilla
   Apple crumble 71
   Banana pancakes 6
   Cashew custard 68
   Chai tea chia pudding 12
   Gluten-free banana bread 78
   Muffins 75
   Nut milk 95
   Whipped creamy coconut 68

Vegetable soup 34
vegetable stock .... *See stock*
vegetables, roasted
    I could cry - creamy soup 59
    Not fast enough five-minute casserole 60
    Resuscitating Thai curry 64
    Right now roast 63
    Suddenly salad 62
vinegar, rice
    Asian style dumplings 27
vinegar, white wine
    Minted potato salad 17
vinegar, wine
    Pork san choy bau 44

W

walnut
    Spicy pumpkin cake 82
Warm your heart - soups **31**
Whipped creamy coconut 68
wine, white
    Sautéed pork with lemon caper sauce 45
    Slow cooked French rillette 55

X

xanthan gum
    Anzac cookies 77
    Low thiol & gluten-free flour 75
    Pumpkin & ginger tart 79

Y

yogurt, coconut
    Banana pancakes 6
    Muffins 75
    Raw raspberry & beetroot no-cheese cake 69
You're sweet enough To temp your guests and delight your taste buds **65**

Z

zucchini
    Chicken stock and bone broths 40
    Low thiol vegetable stock 16
    Thai-style fish curry 41
    Vegetable soup 34
    Zucchini noodles with avocado pesto 22
Zucchini noodles with avocado pesto 22

www.ingramcontent.com/pod-product-compliance
Lightning Source LLC
Chambersburg PA
CBHW040728020526
44107CB00085B/2926